THE REN.
AMERICAN MEDICINE

A Century of New Learning and Caring

To John Paton – a friend without whose skillful help this book would have remained a manuscript – thank you. John

Alan C. Mermann

Alan

University Press of America,® Inc.
Lanham · New York · Oxford

Copyright © 2001 by
University Press of America,® Inc.
4720 Boston Way
Lanham, Maryland 20706

12 Hid's Copse Rd.
Cumnor Hill, Oxford OX2 9JJ

Library of Congress Cataloging-in-Publication Data

Mermann, Alan C.
The renaissance of American medicine : a century of new
learning and caring / Alan C. Mermann.
p.   cm.
Includes bibliographical references and index.
1. Medicine—United States—History. 2. Physicians—United States—
History. 3. Medical care—United States—History. I. Title.
[DNLM: 1. Physicians—United States—Biography. 2. History of
Medicine, 19th Cent.—United States. 3. History of Medicine,
20th Cent.—United States. WZ 140 AA1M566r   2000]
RA395.A3 M464   2000   610'.973—dc21   00-046672 CIP

ISBN 0-7618-1864-2 (cloth : alk. ppr.)
ISBN 0-7618-1865-0 (pbk. : alk. ppr.)

This book is dedicated to

John Harley Warner
and
Frederic L. Holmes
with
admiration and gratitude
for
their teaching and encouragement

Contents

Preface

This study represents a personal search of the past for instruction and enlightenment about the present. We have been warned that ignoring the past can lead to repeating it. However, reliving some events and relationships in the past can be a sheer delight for many of us. The excitement associated with discoveries in laboratories and in minds, the awe and wonder of being present to revelations of truth and beauty, and the humility before genius and invention: we might well wish to have been there.

My interest in the history of medicine, as in history in general, has been developed and sustained by my experiences as a physician for fifty-odd years, an ordained minister for twenty, and a fascinated observer of my world. I am fortunate to have had the opportunities to pursue studies in a variety of fields of inquiry, opening up concepts and ideas previously unknown to me. Of even greater importance has been an evolving awareness of the vastness of the unexplored continents of imagination and thought. The more we pursue any disciplined academic field of study, the more we are made aware of the deficiencies in our knowledge, the dubious nature of much of our reasoning, and the shaky, often false, foundations of many of our assumed convictions.

This study examines in some detail the accepted bases of medical practice in the United States in the century between 1830 and 1920, a time that I call the renaissance of medicine in this country. The focus is upon individual physicians who, observing their times with some care, saw the need for change, for education, for intelligent criticism of method and professional status. These were years of impressive scientific advances, and the responses of the medical profession were often resistant to the opportunities for improvement that were offered.

The study of history is a sober reminder that we must keep in mind that we shall be judged in the future by our odd ideas, our erroneous conclusions, our absurd assurances of the obvious correctness of our interpretations. Today we smile, or we shudder with disbelief, when we read of diagnoses, theories of etiology, and accepted therapies of the past. Perhaps an imagined future study of our history should make us cautious of our judgments about our present knowledge and practice.

A final concern of mine that applies to almost all areas of human intellectual activity is our propensity to believe that, in describing what we see, we are explaining it. There is, finally, no known scientific explanation for what we are and see. We can describe what we see, we can document the reactions we observe between molecules or persons, and we can photograph the supernovas; but we do not know why they are as they are. Final explanations elude human understanding. Thus, we study history to inform us of our past so that we remain humble in the present, even as we lay the groundwork for the future.

Alan C. Mermann
New Haven, Connecticut
July 1, 2000

Introduction

The history of medical practice in the United States is a fascinating, complex, and intricate story about a profession that evolved over time in a pattern that mirrored closely the national political, economic, and social histories. The importance and the intricacies of two intimately related aspects of any profession - education and the techniques of practice - are demonstrated clearly when we study the training and the practices of American physicians during the past tumultuous 250 years.

Since changes in the ways any profession is practiced do not just appear but are reflections of the thoughts and the actions of individuals active in that profession, this book will present biographical studies of physicians whom I consider representative and definitive of the remarkable period - 1830 to 1920 - when American Medicine came of age. Obviously, in a century so filled with astounding events and personalities, my selection of subjects for study is both limited and quite personal. The physicians I have chosen do present, however, many of the personal traits, even idiosyncrasies of character, that work for change and, we hope, improvement in the human condition.

These physicians were educated in the period in our national narrative that began in the decades prior to the Civil War and ends after World War I. While we certainly know the influences of devastating natural catastrophes on our human history, most events are set into motion by persons. Specific actions, writings, works of art and drama, and spoken words are the driving forces behind changes that we acknowledge as important in our long history. For it is the work of individuals who, with their words and acts, initiate societal, scientific, and political movements and social and personal philosophies that change our futures. Unrecognized though they may be at the moment, the commitments and the power of individuals change our world.

One of the remarkable characteristics of our history is its cyclical pattern: at a time when all seems to be calm and serene, forces are already in motion to upset the current 'Era of Good Feeling.' At times of disruption and confusion when hopes for a better world seem nonexistent, there are persons with visions, with expectations, with confidence in the correctness of their plans and the strength to persist who are working for change or renewal. Revolutions - violent or peaceful - have their origins, and are in process, long before they occur. So, too, with our history of medicine. In the very years of the nineteenth century - years of bad practice, no licensing, negligible educational resources, and widespread quackery - there were women and men who were thinking, studying, planning, and teaching ways to change American medical practice. The stories of some of these physicians are the centerpiece of these essays.

To set the stage for my study of these persons who called for and effected changes in both the science and the practice of medicine, I will present, in the first chapter, an historical survey of the status of medical education and practice in the United States in the Colonial/Revolutionary Era. I will begin with a brief appreciation of a famous Massachusetts Bay Colony minister - Cotton Mather - who practiced medicine. His life, both ministerial and medical, will place us in the position of understanding the status of medical practice in those early days of the seventeenth and eighteenth centuries. The colonies were struggling to survive in an inhospitable land far from the assurances of the mother country. Soon would come the years, not only of the growth of population and expansion of territory, but also the years when medical education became established as a reality in America. The importance of the teachings of three European doctors - Thomas Sydenham, William Cullen, and Herman Boerhaave - will be outlined as the founding of the first American medical school is described.

The Jacksonian Democratic Era is the background for the second chapter that will present the decline and decay in medical practice in the United States. It is one of the enduring paradoxes of the history of medicine that, coincident with medical practice reaching its nadir in the United States in the middle years of the nineteenth century, there was a renewed flow of American physicians to Europe to learn the latest in the emerging sciences and practices of medicine. These years saw the awakening, the renaissance that began with this resurgence of studies by American students and practitioners in Paris, Vienna, and Germany. American medicine would be renewed.

Subsequent chapters will examine the professional lives of some men and women who, in the succeeding nineteenth century, made distinctive contributions to the slowly evolving profession of medicine as it adjusted to the new sciences, both physical and social. These physicians, in their studies, practices, and public efforts, introduced ideas and concepts that would significantly change the practice of medicine and bring new understanding of the impact of environment, social custom, prejudice, and belief on the health of the people. Later, I will use the years that witnessed the Reform Movement and subsequently the period of the Progressive Era to complete this brief tour of the remarkable remodeling of American medicine.

These were years of astounding transformation in the nation, ranging from early Puritan towns in New England to the settlement of the West, from Jamestown to Pittsburgh, from the Gold Rush to Wall Street, from slavery to women's suffrage. These were years also of emerging biological sciences such as physiology and pathology, and the radical re-thinking of our place in the world of nature introduced into our self-understanding by Darwin's theory of natural selection and evolution. They were also years of cults and quackery, of the introduction of anesthesia and homeopathy, and of a new confidence in the ability of Nature to heal. It was the time, also, of the revelations of the remarkable new knowledge in the physical sciences of chemistry and physics that introduced radical alterations in our understanding of disease processes and attempts to find rational methods for treating them. Never again would we see ourselves in the same ways as before. These physical sciences presented challenging, even threatening, prospects for established doctrine and practice of medicine.

Central to understanding the stories of these earlier times and of these lives is the necessity of setting aside our easy criticisms of the beliefs and actions of doctors 150 years ago based upon our current knowledge. It is important both to see and to place ourselves, as best we can, in the world that these physicians, patients, and students knew, and acknowledge the fact that they were intelligent, well-read, thoughtful persons who were acting on what they accepted as known, as correct about themselves and their world. We learn very little about ourselves by hasty judgments made on the past. Only the future years will decide on the accuracy of the knowledge we profess to possess and the wisdom of our analyses and our behaviors.

These years were replete with conflicts and misunderstandings that would, as new knowledge and experiences raised questions about a revered past, open the possibilities of health and hope for America. I will close with an appraisal of the new medical educational ventures described in a landmark study, the Flexner Report of 1910 that summarized the state of medical education and practice as the twentieth century began. Central to the revival - the renaissance - of American medicine would be new definitions of the qualifications of the medical student, the teacher, and the methods and goals of teaching medicine.

Chapter 1

Medicine in Colonial America

To get some perspective on the degree and the extent of changes in American medicine during the century from 1830 to 1920 I will, in this first chapter, offer an overview of the 'state of the art' of medical practice in the colonial period, the years leading up to the Revolution. These were years of excitement over what seemed unlimited prospects for a new life for many in a new land, as well as years of suffering and loss for many others far from home. In the second chapter I will describe the powerful impact of Jacksonian democracy on medical education and practice, an impact that raised barriers to efforts of the profession to organize and educate its members. The very presence of these barriers challenged some physicians to seek new resources for education and training. These physicians laid the intellectual, sociopolitical, and practical groundwork during the era this book will discuss for the twentieth century that saw American medicine reach its hoped-for excellence.

In the early years of settlement death rates were high, especially in the southern colonies. Statistics from Virginia are terrifying. Wyndam B. Blanton, in his 1930 book, *Medicine in Virginia in the Seventeenth Century,* noted that,

> In the early years at Jamestown [first settled in 1607], before 1618, 1,100 out of 1,700 immigrants perished. . Six hundred and sixty-five died between 1610 and 1618.... Six hundred were left in Virginia.
> After 1618 the number of immigrants increased, averaging more than a thousand a year. But in February 1625 only 1,095 remained out of 7,549. Not one out of six had survived.[1]

This appalling death rate is probably due to a variety of diseases difficult to define accurately today. The evidence from descriptions would suggest the following as major causes of the high mortality: typhoid fever and other dysenteries, yellow fever, plague, malaria, and nutritional deficit disorders such as famine, scurvy and beriberi. Immigrants learned that the summer months were deadly, and winter became the preferred season for traveling to Virginia.

The early settlers in the Massachusetts Bay Colony fared better, not being as subject to the 'agues' - fevers - as their southern fellow immigrants. There were sporadic epidemics of smallpox, scarlet fever, and measles that took a toll; in the northern climate influenza and pneumonia were major causes of death in the winter season. An outstanding cause of death recorded in the port cities was the loss of ships' crews from drowning. Another factor in the marked differences in population growth between the two colonies could be differences in the social status of the immigrants. A very large percentage of Virginia settlers were indentured servants and criminals banned to the colony. In Massachusetts the settlers were primarily persons leaving England for religious reasons: the Pilgrim and Puritan component of early Massachusetts is well known. It may be that education, community cohesion, and a sounder economy offered some protection against nutritional deficiency diseases and accidental deaths.

The most accurate accounts of mortality rates are found in parish records kept by ministers, many of whom detailed deaths by age, race, gender, and probable cause. An excellent example is seen in the records kept by Ezra Stiles, minister of the Second Congregational Church in Newport, Rhode Island in the 1760s. Stiles - later President of Yale College from 1778 to 1795 - was an intellectual man influenced by Enlightenment thought. He declined a belief in a willful and capricious God who punished by inflicting disease and disaster on sinners. Stiles was an avid accountant of mortality, interested in knowing who died in inns, almshouses, boardinghouses or at home. Stiles also used all possible resources for his figures: midwives, physicians, sextons, and those responsible for the care of the poor. James E. Cassedy, in his 1980 essay on church record keeping in *Medicine in Colonial Massachusetts 1620-1820*, wrote,

> By far the largest number of deaths that Stiles recorded each year had occurred at the beginning of life. About one death in every five was of an infant under a year old, while eight or ten additional were stillbirths. The second largest incidence of mortality understandably came at the other end of the life span...with some one out of seven deaths occurring among individuals over sixty.... Stiles also recorded, almost every year, the deaths of two or three mothers in child-bed...In 1764, his informants pinpointed five deaths from consumption and one from cancer.... Year in and year out, the one specific disease which constantly appeared on his lists...was smallpox.[2]

There were very few regular physicians among the early colonists. Nathan Smith Davis, in his 1851 *History of Medical Education and*

Institutions in the United States... commenting on the rarity of physicians in the early years, did note that a "Dr. Samuel Fuller, a regularly educated physician and highly esteemed man, accompanied the first emigrants who landed at Plymouth in 1620." But this was a rarity. Davis continued by stating the obvious reasons for the lack of doctors:

> [N]o man already established in practice on the other side of the Atlantic, would think of leaving it for the hardships, the poverty, and wilds of America; while the absence of all those medical societies and institutions, which constitute so powerful an object to the aspiring ambition of the thoroughly educated student, equally prevented this class from resorting hither.[3]

Physicians unsuccessful in practice or aware of their own inadequacies in education and training were, therefore, those most likely to come to America.

With the small number of physicians in the colonies, care of the sick was frequently in the hands of lay women and men - often referred to as 'domestics' - who professed some knowledge of that care, and knew something about the herbal, chemical, and surgical means of treating persons who sought their help. The traditional distinctions in England among physician, surgeon, and apothecary were lost in the colonies. The physician was the educated person with a university degree; surgeons - often called barber-surgeons - received minimal education, usually as an apprentice. Apothecaries were popular sources of help for those unwilling or unable to find a doctor. With the small number of doctors available to a widely scattered population in thirteen colonies, medical care was difficult to find, usually clustered in the cities and large towns. Physicians - well-dressed gentlemen with the identifiable gold-headed cane - were a rarity.

The Companies that were commercial sponsors of the colonies usually provided some medical help in the persons of surgeons or apothecaries who served their colonies for a specified, and usually brief, time. These professional 'comforters of the sick,' as the Dutch called them, went on to train others in the colonies as an apprentice system was being developed. The apprentice was usually an adolescent boy, often an orphan, who signed an agreement similar to a legal contract, to work with and for a practicing doctor of one kind or another for a specific number of years, often six or seven. This was very similar to the way in which indentured servants were acquired in that time. There was little, if any, distinction between apprenticeship to a doctor, to a cobbler, or to a blacksmith. William Dosite Postell, writing in 1958, described the system.

> Training, as understood at that time, was largely received by the apprenticeship method. Medicine shared in this outlook, and physicians were trained as apprentices. Of the 3500 practitioners in America at the beginning of the Revolution, only 400 held M.D. degrees, and most of them were from foreign universities...anyone could practice medicine and almost everyone did.... The one exception to this in colonial America was the practice of obstetrics, which was still dominated by midwives.[4]

The system was a standard one. The apprentice usually lived in the house of the doctor, carried out menial household tasks, read the doctor's few textbooks, collected fees, and observed the current state of the art, such as it was. At the conclusion of his obligated tenure, the apprentice received a note confirming his training and his abilities that then was filed with the local court. There were no examinations or licensing procedures. In time, those who were apprenticed assumed the role of doctor and took apprentices themselves. It would be years before any effective system would be developed to determine the qualifications of those professing to treat the sick. Some sense of the level of professional skills in the early days of colonization can be grasped by this brief description of the education of seventeenth century American doctors.

New England Clergy-Physicians

Religious persecution in England in the late sixteenth and early seventeenth centuries encouraged the migration of highly educated and trained men, including, of course, clergy dissenting from the Church of England. These ministers were to become important practitioners of medicine in the seventeenth century in New England. There are several factors that placed ministers in the roles of physicians. First, ministers were university graduates, and part of the routine education of all students was lectures on medicine. This material was based largely on the ancient texts of Hippocrates and Galen and required reading ability in Latin and in Greek, skills that barber-surgeons and apothecaries did not possess. This ability to read provided access to medical texts not available to any other colonist except physicians who were in rare supply. Second, universities were the only available source for studying the new sciences that were emerging as the Enlightenment was being born. A fascination with botany was common, with interests in foreign plants and trees fanned by the explorations that began in the fifteenth century. Knowledge of botany was important, of course, because herbal medicines were crucial for medical care and ministers could read the literature needed for treating their flocks. These years of settlement of the Americas by Spanish, Portuguese, Swedish, English, and Dutch explorers coincided with growing interests in natural history and the embryonic sciences of astronomy, mathematics, physics, and chemistry. Genevieve Miller described this time of transition in her 1956 essay.

> After the recovery of the best thought of antiquity, uncorrupted texts of classical authors, men learned to look at nature not only as the Greeks had done, but what was more important, to see it with their own eyes. The discovery and colonization of the New World ran parallel with and was analogous to the discovery and exploration of the whole realm of natural phenomena. There was a reciprocal reaction between the two that molded the character of early modern times in all its cultural manifestations.[5]

The early colonists of Massachusetts Bay interpreted bad events, be they diseases, accidents, or bad weather as God-given punishment for sinful behavior. With the changes secondary to their education and their new knowledge in the study of nature, the clergy, in particular, became caregivers of body as well as of soul. John Winthrop, Sr., the governor of Massachusetts, took it upon himself to obtain medical prescriptions from doctors in England so that he might treat the sick. His son, a famous physician and a governor of Connecticut, received letters from across the colonies seeking advice and assistance in treating various ills. During the smallpox epidemic of 1677-78 the Reverend Thomas Thacher of the Old South Church in Boston printed the first medical document in the colonies, a paper to help victims of the disease. An excellent example of the abilities of the 'clerical physician' is found in Cotton Mather (1663-1728), ordained in 1685 to join his father, Increase Mather, as a minister to Old South Church. He provides a delightful picture of the mixture we find in intelligent persons in all ages: an inquisitive mind locked into the fallacies of his day, and an inner courage to do what seems logical and right for those for whom he accepts responsibility.

Mather was subject to melancholia as a boy and, as an adolescent, tried self-treatment that he read about; his father had a large library and also access to the library of Harvard College, of which he was president. Cotton Mather also had a stammer that he thought would make a career as a preacher impossible. He seriously considered becoming a physician, and held medicine and theology - science and religion - in a careful balance throughout his life. His stammer cleared and he assumed his prominent clerical role. There was only one doctor in Boston with an M.D. degree, Doctor William Douglass who would become wealthy and an enemy of Mather over the question of inoculation against smallpox. Another factor, unfortunately not rare in our history, that played a role in clerical medical ministrations was the tendency of doctors to ignore the social needs of the poor so apparent to the clergy.

Doctors were very reluctant to incorporate any of the new sciences into the 'physic' practiced at the bedside. Mather, however, was interested in the sciences and was elected into the Royal Society in 1713, the year of his publication of a pamphlet on measles. He submitted over one hundred letters to its *Philosophical Transactions,* none of which were published. Mather pursued his interests in the physic of his day and, in 1724, wrote a lengthy treatise on medicine, *Angel of Bethesda.* Also unpublished, it remains a delightful source of information on the beliefs of that day. One medical observation of Mather that seems most prescient for our time is quoted by Beall and Shryock in their 1954 study of Mather: "'the *caustic Salt* in the *Smoke'* of tobacco 'may lay Foundations for Diseases in Millions of unadvised People.'"[6]

Mather was a proponent of what would become preventive medicine. He was in contact with the German Pietists at Halle, incorporating their commitments to medical care of the poor into his own work. In response to the indifference of local physicians, Mather took upon himself the task of introducing inoculation against smallpox when the disease reached Boston in 1721. Reported from China as early as 1700, in 1714 a notice of the practice of inoculation in Turkey was published by the Royal Society. In 1716 Mather wrote to the Society that he heard about inoculation in Africa from his servant, Onesimus. When Mather questioned him whether he had had smallpox, he answered both 'yes' and 'no.' He explained that he had had a small 'operation' that inoculated him with the disease. In a pamphlet written in 1722 on smallpox Mather is quite certain that, in the future, it will be found that the external cause of this dreadful epidemic lies in pathogenic animalculae: referring to smallpox as an invading enemy, he wrote that "many now think this 'an animalculated business.'"[7]

Cotton Mather is a wonderful example of the mixture that we are. A prosecutor in the famous Salem witch trials of 1682, a believer in the strangest of remedies and causes of physical events, he was also an early witness to the coming of the Enlightenment with its confidence in science and reason. He was dedicated to the care of the poor and an example of courage in his pursuit of inoculation despite the powerful opposition of local doctors who, in fact, had his house bombed in 1721 during the smallpox epidemic.

Medical Education

In the first century of colonization opportunities in America to study traditional medicine as practiced in England and Europe did not exist; the first medical college in America was not established until 1765. For those who had the financial means, travel to England, Scotland, or Holland was necessary to find hospital and teaching facilities adequate for training. Three cities were paramount: London, Edinburgh, and Leyden. But it was not the city that drew the students; it was the physicians teaching there. In keeping with my emphasis on the persons who figured strongly in the changes that would take place in medical practice and education, I will present brief biographical sketches of three men in these cities who were outstanding in their time: Thomas Sydenham, William Cullen, and Herman Boerhaave. Two characteristics of these men set the stage for remarkable changes in medical practice. First, they tended to reject classical education in Latin and Greek as taught at Cambridge and Oxford, and the theories inherited from Galen describing the causes of diseases and their treatments; second, they relied on detailed descriptions of the medical histories and observations of their patients' diseases, recording these findings as case-histories that would later become recorded as disease-histories that would provide a firm foundation for teaching students.

Thomas Sydenham

Thomas Sydenham (1624-1689) was a member of a family that played an active military role in establishing the Commonwealth under Cromwell. Sydenham was, in fact, a cavalry officer and was seriously wounded in the Civil War. After the fighting ceased he returned to Oxford to continue his studies, unsure of his future career. On his way to Oxford he met a Dr. Thomas Coxe who was caring for Sydenham's sick brother. In conversation with the doctor, he was encouraged to study medicine. How simply decisions can be made!

Education at the universities was in disarray due to the recent war, and the medical curriculum was antiquated, relying heavily on theories and formal disputations that seemed to have little to do with the care of the sick. A contemporary student of Sydenham wrote, "Physick, says Sydenham, is not to be learned by going to universities, but hee is for taking apprentices; and says one had as good send a man to Oxford to learn shoemaking as practicing physick."[8] While at Oxford Sydenham developed a lasting friendship with Robert Boyle, a leading scientist and a member of the Royal Society. One of the ongoing wonders of this study of biographies is the discovery that Sydenham, a close friend of several prominent members of the Royal Society responsible for the new sciences of chemistry and physics evolving in the seventeenth century (Boyle, Hooke, Willis), had no confidence in scientific investigation as a way of understanding the human body and its diseases.

After three years of desultory study at Oxford Sydenham married in 1655 and set up his medical practice near swampy St. James's Park. The close proximity of this swamp afforded him a considerable clientele of fever patients, and he began to classify fevers in several categories: continuous, intermittent, and smallpox. Encouraged by Boyle, he set about studying London epidemics that included diseases we know as typhoid and typhus fevers, malaria, measles, and smallpox. Sydenham described and named the disease, scarlet fever. This streptococcal infection was often followed by rheumatic fever; the associated arthritis in its varied forms was to become an ongoing interest for him. His name is also attached to another occasional sequela of rheumatic fever, chorea, known in former times as St. Vitus' Dance. In 1676 Sydenham published his major work, *Medical Observations,* a collection of essays that became a major educational resource for physicians in America and Europe.

In a detailed letter to another physician, William Cole, Sydenham rejected the accepted doctrine that hysteria was a female disorder due to a 'wandering uterus.' He found that men were as susceptible to the psychological symptoms as women, and labeled the male disorder as hypochondriasis. Another aspect of his medical practice not accepted by the profession for many years was his willingness to observe and document the course of a disease before attempting treatments that were so often futile. Kenneth Dewhurst, in his 1966 biography of Sydenham, wrote, "Sydenham's treatment was never rigid or dogmatic: sometimes he omitted medication altogether, simply leaving the patient to the care of 'the prince and pattern of physicians - Time.'"[9] As part of his discontent with university education Sydenham was a major proponent of learning medicine from a preceptor as an apprentice rather than attending lectures. In an interesting anecdote Richard Blackmore commented on Sydenham's distrust of contemporary medical teaching. "When one day I asked him to advise me what 'Books I should read to qualify me for Practice,'" wrote Blackmore, "'he replied, Read *Don Quixote,* it is a very good Book, I read it still.'"[10]

The characteristic of the medical practice of Sydenham that was to become central to future teaching was his insistence upon documenting detailed descriptions of disease. In this practice he relied upon the teaching of Hippocrates that emphasized the need for scrupulous descriptions of the manifestations of diseases on patients. Although he accepted the ancient humoral theory of pathogenesis, he easily set it aside when his evaluation of the patient did not corroborate it. The evidence of experience was the deciding factor in both diagnosis and treatment. An example of this was his immediate acceptance of Peruvian bark - quinine - for the treatment of intermittent fever, a condition we know as malaria. If Peruvian bark worked, it was to be used.

In Sydenham's practical understanding of medicine, the teachings of Francis Bacon about experimental methods were central. A close friend who was supportive and admiring of Sydenham's work was John Locke, a physician renowned for his writings on political philosophy and the nature of the human mind in understanding reality. Locke, in a letter to Dr. Thomas Molyneux, commented on the need to document the workings of Nature. He wrote, "So there is nothing left for a Physician to do, but to observe well, and so by Analogy, argue the like Cases, and thence make himself Rules of Practice: and he that is this way most sagacious, will, I imagine, make the best Physician...."[11]

Dewhurst, commenting on Sydenham, noted that this physician's reputation depended

> upon the general clinical principles which guided his own practice of medicine and illustrated his writings. Sydenham's revival of the Hippocratic method of studying the natural history of diseases by making a series of accurate and detailed observations set the clinical pattern of future progress.[12]

Herman Boerhaave

Herman Boerhaave (1668-1738) was probably the best known and most respected physician of the eighteenth century in Europe and America. The son of a clergyman, he studied philosophy, mathematics, and metaphysics, taking his first degree in theology in 1690. He did not follow his father's calling, but went on to study botany and chemistry, finally taking a degree in medicine in 1693. A commentary on his brilliance and on the state of medical education in his time is the fact that he never attended lectures, preferring to study the Hippocratic writings at home. At the university there was no teaching in the sciences; almost all instruction was done by lectures on theories. To get some understanding of the status of medical education and training at that time, G. A. Lindeboom, in his comprehensive 1968 biography of Boerhaave, wrote,

> [B]efore Boerhaave's appearance practical medicine was in a state of confusion and often not more that a precarious empiricism.... Knowledge of anatomy and pathology was only poorly integrated into medicine...Clinical medicine was not well developed, and good bedside teaching was exceedingly rare. Moreover there was an obvious lack of reliable textbooks. Hence, there was a lifetime's work for a man with keen insight into the momentous needs of theoretical and practical medicine and of medical education. Such a man made his appearance in Boerhaave.[13]

Boerhaave probably did attend the anatomy dissections that became available to the public. He began his practice in Leyden, the university city that became the Mecca for men seeking the best medical training available in that century.

Boerhaave read widely in all categories of literature. His reading of Isaac Newton's *Principia,* published in 1687, awakened him to the new sciences and he became a devoted student of chemistry and physics. Boerhaave was highly intelligent and he refused to fall into any one system of thought in his time. He was an ardent admirer of Sydenham, recently dead, whose writings were in full force at the time. It is a commentary on Boerhaave's selective reading that he complimented Sydenham on his descriptions of disease based upon observation and not on theory, while fully accepting the sciences that Sydenham refused to acknowledge. These were years of exciting discussion as the writings of Spinoza (1632-1677) and Descartes (1596-1650) stimulated new thought and experiment in strenuous efforts to understand the workings of the natural world, in particular the human body and its functions and diseases.

In 1701 Boerhaave was appointed to the faculty at Leyden, beginning his illustrious career as physician, investigator, and teacher. His lifelong interest in botany encouraged the development of a superior garden at the University greatly supplemented by seeds brought from abroad by the captains of the Dutch ships that traveled the seas. The garden was a permanent fixture in his life. He was a man of wide interests, open to new ideas and new concepts. He persisted in avoiding all attempts to create theories about disease and healing. As with Sydenham, he relied heavily on observation at the bedside and documentation of the course of diseases. He became a major support for physicians in later years who placed growing confidence in the power of Nature to cure, seeing the doctor as one who could damage as well as heal. Using a magnifying glass to examine the eye, Boerhaave gave what were probably the first lectures on ophthalmology. He also used a thermometer to record the body temperature of his patients.

As one would expect, Boerhaave wrote about medicine in its many modes. He published a two-volume edition of the important *Fabrica* of Vesalius, the anatomy text that revolutionized our understanding of the human body, and, with Sydenham, dismissed Galen as a source of medical knowledge. His major work, the *Institutes of Medicine,* would remain the standard textbook for years. He wrote botanical studies, a book on aphorisms, a study of venereal diseases, and disputations that countered popular Cartesian arguments. Boerhaave had an elegant interior life of the mind that joined his education and his reflections on science and medicine and supported him through the vicissitudes of a busy and dedicated life.

In a collection of his lectures on the history of medicine given to seniors at Northwestern University Medical School in the years 1892-1896, Nathan Smith Davis wrote this evaluation of Boerhaave.

> As a man of great erudition, close observation and logical reasoning, he had few equals among contemporaries; and as a general practitioner and teacher of medicine he gained a wider reputation and had more influence than any other physician of the eighteenth century. His advice was sought by all classes of people, from those highest in authority to the common laborer and he insisted on giving each his turn, regardless of rank or wealth.[14]

Leyden became a magnet both for practicing American physicians and for those who, apprenticed to doctors, realized that they needed more education. The central role of European training was known and appreciated.

William Cullen

William Cullen (1710-1790) was a Scottish physician who had a unique role in the early development of medical education in America. In 1755 he was appointed professor of chemistry and medicine at the University of Edinburgh; his academic career developed nicely and 1773 he became the sole professor of physic (medicine) at Edinburgh and First Physician to the King of Scotland, positions he held until his death seventeen years later. He is of interest to us, not only because of his outstanding personal career as doctor and teacher, but also because of his influence on the first medical school in the colonies founded in Philadelphia in 1765. His teaching also provides a view of a method of medical education called 'system' that was to become the focus of serious debate in the nineteenth century.

The word, system, would acquire a bad name in future years as the new sciences allied to physiology developed and became central to a new understanding of medical practice. In the eighteenth century, however, as a response to the Enlightenment, the assurance of innate powers of Reason in the human mind encouraged a confidence that speculation and informed thought could create intellectual frameworks that would help us understand the complex order of Nature, making it comprehensible and manageable. 'System' was, then, an attempt to improve the practice of medicine by delineating the fundamentals of diagnosis and treatment by reasoned thought. The problem was that there was little, if any, rational basis for most systems of medicine, and exactly opposite theories were proposed based upon the same observations and conjectures.

William Cullen received his education at the University of Glasgow over a period of fourteen years. After finishing his general studies at the age of twenty and serving as an apprentice apothecary-surgeon, he took a position for a year as surgeon on a merchant ship visiting the West Indies. He returned to practice medicine, went back to Glasgow for more formal education, took medical classes at Edinburgh, and finally received his M.D. degree from Glasgow - a school of questionable medical standing at the time - in 1740. In 1755 he moved to Edinburgh to begin his illustrious career.

There are two aspects of Cullen's career that are important for setting the stage for our study of the renaissance in American medicine in the nineteenth century: 1), his personal characteristics as a doctor and a teacher and, 2), his intellectual system for teaching medicine.

First, Cullen was a beloved teacher who devoted some forty years to lecturing and demonstrating his craft. He invited students to his home and was pleased to discuss personal as well as scholarly concerns with them; he treated sick students and the poor without charging fees, and was readily available to other physicians for consultation. A colleague, Dr. James Anderson, wrote,

> Dr. Cullen's professional knowledge was always great, and his manner of lecturing singularly clear and intelligible, lively, and entertaining; and to his patients, his conduct in general, as a physician, was so pleasing, his address so affable and engaging, and his manner so open, so kind, and so regulated by pecuniary considerations, that it was impossible for those who had occasion to call for his medical assistance, ever to be satisfied on any

future occasion without it. He became the friend and companion of every family he visited.[15]

Cullen was a cautious prescriber and treater, preferring moderation in the use of drugs, dietary modification, and procedures such as bleeding. His reputation as a physician spread throughout Britain and Europe and he developed an extensive consultation practice by mail. There are some 3000 letters on record that document the extent of his careful and considered advice given both to other physicians and to patients over many years. We may think it quite odd that one would diagnose and prescribe by mail, but it was a natural response to the practice methods of the time. The history of the symptoms of the patient, facts such as diet, season of the year, geographic location and occupation, the pulse rate and a cursory examination comprised a visit to the doctor. The stethoscope had not yet been invented, temperatures were not taken, and there were no laboratory tests other than examining the urine visually and by odor.

Second, Cullen's 'system' of medicine was not as rigid as we might expect from the writings of others. He used the word, system, as a signal to orient one's thoughts in an integrated manner around available knowledge in order to make some sense of experience. He was a firm believer in collecting facts: he was a botanist and a chemist in his day. He also required as much information about his patients as possible, including post-mortem findings, if available. He also placed importance on the effects of the mind on the body and was the first physician to use the word, neuroses, to describe what he took to be psychological symptoms. 'System,' for Cullen, seemed to be a way of bringing current knowledge together so as to make some sense of diseases and their treatments. He advocated systematic study and teaching as the way to hold together what was known in his day. Perhaps the key to understanding Cullen's concept of system can be read in a 1750 letter to a former student, Balfour Russell, about two kinds of study.

> The first kind should be for perfecting yourself in some system.... The system may be what you please...a system which you make for yourself out of all of them. You will not find it possible to separate practice from theory altogether; and therefore, if you have a mind to begin with the theory, I have no objection.[16]

The reader picks up, in Cullen's *P.S.* to the letter, his perennial interest in learning.

Let me beg of you to have no scruple with regard to what you should write. I do not expect new discoveries in every line, and I would rather bear with twenty old and common things, than miss one new fact or observation.[17]

The first six professors at the Medical School of the College of Philadelphia, founded in 1765, received their medical degrees from Edinburgh. John Morgan, William Shippen, Jr., Benjamin Rush, Adam Kuhn, Philip Syng Physick, and George Wistar would be outstanding leaders in their time and place, ensuring the growth of medical education and improved clinical practice in the colonies. The elite College of Physicians of Philadelphia, founded in 1787, comprised about half of the practicing doctors in the city, and could count one-third of them as having trained in Edinburgh. For this group the teaching of William Cullen would be both practiced and cherished. In his 1993 essay on the influence of Cullen on American medicine, John M. O'Donnell wrote,

Cullen, then, was a teacher with a persuasive pedagogy and warm personality who befriended many of his American pupils and who influenced them by force of example.... He developed a model of clinical teaching and a style of professional conduct that were deliberately and at times unconsciously replicated in North America.... Cullen's direct and indirect influence was indeed considerable.[18]

Beginning in the sixteenth century, public anatomy dissection of the human body became a popular entertainment in Italy, in Holland, and later in England and Scotland. Anatomy theaters were built and the public was invited - at an admission fee - to witness the dissections. In England, passage of the Murder Act of 1732 gave the bodies of executed criminals to the anatomists, linking destruction of the body to loss of the soul as final punishment for the crimes they had committed.

An outstanding colleague of Cullen was Alexander Monro, professor of anatomy at the University of Edinburgh. Within a few years of his beginning to teach, he had about 150 persons attending his lectures: surgeons, medical students, and - the largest part of his audience - the public. In 1739 Monro compiled a list of the uses of anatomy, a grading system that instructs us on eighteenth century categories of understanding the place of the human being in the created world. First on the list of uses was natural theology, not surgery. In fact, surgery was fifth on the list after philosophy, law, and art. The human body held many religious meanings for people, and was shrouded in a rich tapestry of symbol and ritual. Early modern anatomy served broad cultural purposes far beyond learning what the body looked like inside.

In these former times, the anatomy theater was regarded by its viewers as a moral theater, a place where emotions were stirred. The feelings described by observers of these eighteenth century anatomists were those associated with death: awe, pity, and compassion. Although the categories have changed over time, the mystery and wonder of the human body in all its functions continue to amaze and delight us, even bewildering us in its complexity and beauty.

America's First Medical Schools

By the early years of the eighteenth century the colonies had grown in population and in economic stability. The 'starving time' was over and America became attractive to many persons in the professional as well as artisan classes. Physicians emigrated from England, Scotland, and Europe who demonstrated training that was obviously superior to the apprentice system prominent in America. This observation persuaded American physicians to go to Europe to upgrade their training, if they could afford it. Another observation that recommended training abroad was the very obvious differences between the skills of British and American doctors so apparent during the Anglo-French Wars that occurred, off and on, between 1689 and 1763, preceding the Revolution. Surgery in particular, with its base in anatomical dissection, pointed up the education that was missing in the colonies.

Another missing component of medical training in America was a lack of education in the natural sciences. In his 1956 study, *The Pursuit of Science in Revolutionary America 1735-1789,* Brooke Hindle commented on the prominence of physicians in ongoing studies in the natural sciences. A significant contribution to their interests was the education they received abroad.

> This prominence of physicians in natural history was no accident but resulted from the medical training of that day which afforded an introduction to the study of the sciences of nature. At the progressive schools of Padua, Leyden, and Edinburgh and in the great hospitals of the city of London, medical students took formal courses in botany, in chemistry, and in anatomy - sometimes including comparative anatomy.... many of the trained physicians who emigrated to the colonies, went there after having studied medicine on the continent.[19]

This influx of scientifically educated doctors into the colonies not only encouraged American doctors to study abroad; it provided evidence to the public and to city and college officials that there was a profound need to improve American medical education. Another result that caused a permanent alteration in education was the close ties that were formed between American doctors and important scientific organizations such as The Royal Society, stimulating an impressive and lasting correspondence on scientific issues, a relationship that survived the Revolution. The time was appropriate for establishing formal education programs - medical colleges - that would provide the education and training essential to a new and rapidly developing country soon to become a nation.

The first medical school in the American colonies was established in 1765 as part of the College of Philadelphia. Founded by Benjamin Franklin, the College - later to become the University of Pennsylvania - was not primarily interested in training men for the ministry, but aimed its education at providing 'useful learning.' Integral to the educational curriculum offered was using the English language, including courses in the sciences, and 'practical' teaching in subjects such as mathematics and geography. Two men were instrumental in the formation of the medical school of Philadelphia, John Morgan and William Shippen, Jr.

John Morgan began his medical apprenticeship to an outstanding physician, John Redman, at the age of fifteen. During his six-year term with Redman, Morgan attended the College of Philadelphia, receiving his A.B. with its first class in 1757. Morgan served briefly as a surgeon during the French and Indian War; he then decided to study abroad. In London he visited hospitals and made important friends, but decided to go to Edinburgh where he received his M.D. degree in 1763. Morgan then left for Europe where he took the 'Grand Tour' making still more influential friends. In Paris in 1764 he wrote a lengthy lecture, *Discourse upon the Institution of Medical Schools in America,* that would be instrumental in providing the groundwork for founding the medical school at the College of Philadelphia, accomplished in 1765. Morgan was subsequently appointed professor of the theory and practice of medicine.

William Shippen, Jr., a graduate of the College of New Jersey (later Princeton) was a friend of Morgan. After his apprenticeship with his father he went to Edinburgh, where Morgan subsequently matriculated. Both men discussed the possibilities of a medical school in Philadelphia and would work together to establish it. Shippen returned to Philadelphia in 1762 and began a series of public anatomical lectures with a collection of anatomical drawings presented to him by Dr. John Fothergill a prominent Quaker physician in London who was supportive of efforts to establish a medical school in the colonies.

Shippen was appointed professor of anatomy and surgery in 1765 and the school was off and running, graduating its first class of ten students in 1768. One of the graduates was Benjamin Rush, a former student at Edinburgh destined to become professor of chemistry at Philadelphia and achieve a nationwide reputation for his insistence on bloodletting as a central therapy for almost all diseases.

An important component of the education at Philadelphia was access to clinical teaching at the Pennsylvania Hospital founded in 1751. Thomas Bond was physician to the hospital and offered clinical lectures at the new school. He was an early and insistent advocate of the centrality of bedside teaching, convinced that lectures were insufficient, and textbooks of limited value for the proper practice of medicine. The medical school preferred students who were college graduates, but accepted those with an adequate knowledge of Latin, philosophy and mathematics. Course requirements for a B.M. were anatomy, chemistry, theory and practice of physic, and materia medica. A year of clinical work at the Pennsylvania Hospital was required. Originally the College offered both the B.M. and M.D., the latter requiring additional course work and a thesis. When it became apparent that few men returned for this degree, the baccalaureate degree was discontinued and graduates received an M.D. degree.

New York was the next city to welcome a medical school. Samuel Bard, son of a prominent New York physician, was also a student at Edinburgh. Learning of the intentions of Shippen and Morgan to establish a school in Philadelphia, Bard proposed the same idea when he returned after receiving his degree from Edinburgh in 1765. By 1767 he had gathered a faculty and the King's College Medical School opened that year, and graduated its first class in May 1769. In his commencement address Bard spoke to the need for a hospital to offer the necessary clinically oriented bedside training for students. Funds subsequently raised provided the means to build The New York Hospital. This new school, the second in America, would eventually become the College of Physicians and Surgeons of Columbia University.

Boston was the next city to have a medical school. John Warren, a graduate of Harvard College in 1771, studied medicine under his brother, Joseph, who was fatally wounded at the Battle of Bunker Hill. Appointed a surgeon by George Washington, John Warren was senior surgeon in the military hospital in Cambridge, and took part in the military campaigns in New Jersey and Pennsylvania. Returning to Boston in 1777, he married, and resumed his post as senior surgeon at Cambridge. A medical club was formed that met at the Green Dragon tavern. At its meeting on May 14, 1780, Warren proposed the creation of a medical school. His proposal was coolly received, but he persisted and, in correspondence with Benjamin Rush in Philadelphia, he gathered detailed information on that school. In November 1782 his formal proposal to the Harvard Corporation was accepted. Warren was appointed professor of anatomy and surgery and two other appointments were made: Benjamin Waterhouse professor of theory and practice, and Aaron Dexter professor of chemistry and materia medica. The following year explicit plans for the school were published that outlined the needs for the medical school as a critical resource for the proper teaching of medicine based upon the sciences and the skills of the best teachers and materials. The Corporation voted to provide a library, anatomical preparations, and a 'theatre' for demonstrations. The Corporation also promised to ask the Legislature for permission to use the bodies of executed criminals and suicides for dissection. Although the school would apparently accept all applicants, undergraduates would only be admitted after two years of study. The standards that were set seem appropriately high for the time and the school was off to a good start.

Nathan Smith, a graduate of Harvard who also studied at Edinburgh, helped organize a medical school at Dartmouth College in 1797. The University of Transylvania in Kentucky opened its medical school in 1802, and Baltimore had its medical school by 1807. All in all, by 1813 there were seven medical colleges chartered and in operation in the United States.

Commentary

On paper, the story of these early medical schools sounds impressive and promising. And, for a beginning it was a hopeful enterprise. But it is important to note some of the negative aspects of these schools that would pose problems for the future. A central issue was the novel demographics of this new nation. Essentially a frontier society widely dispersed over a large area from Maine to Georgia, cities were far apart and transportation could be formidable. Travel to and from the cities - the location of the medical colleges - was difficult. The rural nature of life made the accumulation of money for tuition and room and board a problem for many prospective students who would prefer the apprenticeship system with a local doctor whose credentials, however, might be highly suspect.

The instruction offered in these schools was also subject to criticism. The 'professors' were not of the caliber of the teachers at Leyden, London, Padua, or Edinburgh. They were, instead, young men in their twenties who had studied for a few years at these renowned schools. Also, their teaching was primarily from their notes taken at lectures by their mentors, and lacked the necessary support of personal experience in practice, be it anatomical, therapeutic, or at the bedside. Although these young instructors were committed to their teaching, they often lacked the power and the enthusiasm of a Cullen, Boerhaave, or Hunter. The result was frequent disappointment at the quality of the education offered.

Another problem these new schools faced was widespread public opposition to dissection of human bodies by students. This was obviously a problem for these schools, and the common practice of 'body snatching' was alarming to the general populace. Several riots are recorded in the 1780s in response to robbing the graves of the deceased. However, it was a time of new beginnings, both in medicine and as a nation. And these new beginnings - both political and medical - were created by persons, by individual men who held to a vision that showed a new concept of the future for their country and for their professions. The brief biographical studies of these men is important for grasping the impact that individuals can have on altering the course of our history as it unfolds before us. History is an account of what women and men do as they foresee possibilities for them and those who will follow them.

As the nineteenth century arrived there were two different paths that would be followed. For some the new time was the beginning of reform. In his 1976 study of the early years of medical education, Martin Kaufman wrote,

Although the early medical schools had problems acquiring cadavers for dissection and demonstrations and although the colleges' existence seemed precarious at times, such as during the doctors' riot of 1788, the schools at Philadelphia, New York, and Boston were the start of a great reform movement, a movement that was to be continued in the early nineteenth century with the establishment of similar schools throughout the ever-expanding United States.[20]

As we will see, the new century would not be one of any consistency in reform. The new schools established in the United States would leave much to be desired as sources of proper education in medicine. Genevieve Miller, pointing to this coming time, wrote,

The Revolutionary War closed both medical colleges [Philadelphia and New York] temporarily, and it is regrettable that the fine example set by these schools and by Harvard, where a medical faculty was created in 1783, was not rigorously followed in the subsequent development of medical education in the new nation. Instead the absence of both professional and governmental enforcement of adequate standards, the growing need for more physicians for the expanding population, and the predominantly commercial spirit created an environment favorable to the growth of independent proprietary schools that were the most characteristic American medical institution of the 19th century.[21]

These two quotations point to a basic conviction - an historical assumption - that I will stress: at the very moment when current events support one understanding of the direction that history will take, contrary forces are working toward an opposite goal. As the nineteenth century opened there was optimism for the future of medical education in the United States with the emergence of new medical schools. These schools were originally allied to major colleges that would provide the intellectual, as well as the financial, support for the development of elite and competent educational and training environments. Americans could expect, then, top quality physicians to provide the best care. The next chapter will take us into a different medical world.

---

[1]Blanton, Wyndham B., *Medicine in Virginia in the Seventeenth Century*, Richmond, The William Byrd Press, 1930, 33-34.
[2]Cassedy, James H., "Church Record-Keeping and Public Health in Early New England," in *Medicine in Colonial Massachusetts 1620-1820*, Boston, The Colonial Society of Massachusetts, 1980, 258-259.
[3]Davis, N.S., *History of Medical Education and Institutions in the United States*, Chicago, S.C. Griggs & Co., 1841, 14, 17-18.
[4]Postell, William Dosite, "Medical Education and Medical Schools in Colonial America," *International Record of Medicine*: 171:(June 1958), 365.
[5]Miller, Genevieve, "Medical Education in the American Colonies," *Journal of Medical Education*, 31:2 (February 1956), 83.
[6]Beall, Jr., Otho T., and Shryock, Richard H., *Cotton Mather*, Baltimore, The Johns Hopkins Press, 1954, 51.
[7]Ibid., 113.
[8]Dewhurst, Kenneth, *Dr. Thomas Sydenham (1624-1689): His Life and Original Writings*, Berkeley and Los Angeles, University of California Press, 1966, 17.
[9]Ibid., 47.

[10] Ibid., 49.

[11]Ibid., 189.

[12]Ibid., 59.

[13]Lindeboom, G. A., *Herman Boerhaave: The Man and his Work,* London, Methuen & CO. LTD, 1968, 9.

[14]Davis, Nathan Smith, *History of Medicine with the Code of Medical Ethics,* Chicago, Cleveland Press, 1903, 92.

[15] Thomson, John, *An Account of the Life, Lectures, and Writings of William Cullen, M.D.,* vol. I, Edinburgh and London, William Blackwood and Sons, 1859, 121.

[16] Ibid., 130.

[17] Ibid., 131.

[18]O'Donnell, John M., "Cullen's influence on American medicine," *William Cullen and the Eighteenth Century Medical World,* ed. A. Diog, J.P.S. Ferguson, I.A. Milne and R. Passmore, Edinburgh, Edinburgh University Press, 1993, 243.

[19]Hindle, Brooke, *The Pursuit of Science in Revolutionary America 1735-1789,* Chapel Hill, The University of North Carolina Press, 1956, 36-37.

[20]Kaufman, Martin, *American Medical Education: The Formative Years,1765-1910,* Westport, Ct., Greenwood Press, 32.

[21]Miller, Genevieve, *op. cit.,* 94.

Chapter 2

Years of Conflict and Change

The century from the 1790s to the 1890s was an era of harsh conflict and profound change, not only in medicine but in the social and political structure of the nation. Of course, the centerpiece of conflict was the Civil War, a horrendous experience that effected influences on all aspects of American life, some of which persist to this day. The opening of the West to development with all of its consequences for the people and for the land, massive immigration from Europe, the slow but persistent progress in the physical sciences, and the evolution of both the democratic process and a rising social consciousness - all these make the century a fascinating and instructive study. This century is a stark illustration of the coexistence of powerful and opposing forces that, only vaguely recognized at the time, determine the course our history will take. Since events are not created out of thin air, but by persons, I will center my study on some of the women and men who represent these opposing theories and convictions. The identity of the profession of medicine would be altered both for physicians and their patients, and unwelcome competitors in the healing arts would appear. I will discuss several key topics that illustrate the antagonisms in this century that, under the tutelage of the physicians I will discuss, led to the re-creation of American medicine.

Years of Decline

The first medical schools, established in the colonies along the Atlantic seaboard, were associated with colleges: Philadelphia, New York, Harvard, Dartmouth, Maryland, and Yale. While the original plans had called for two degrees, an M.B. that would be followed seven years later by an M.D., this did not happen. Within a few years the M.B. was discarded and the M.D. became the degree earned, unfortunately with less education required than the original M.B. After the War of 1812 there was a proliferation of medical schools across the country, particularly in rural areas. They would be known as proprietary medical schools because they were 'owned' by the physicians who created them and had them licensed under state laws.

The result was an astounding proliferation of these schools: by 1876 there were sixty-four medical schools, and by 1900, 151. There were a number of reasons for both the decline in training at the college-related schools and the emergence of the proprietary ones.

1. The rapid expansion of the frontier to the West made transportation to eastern cities difficult, and the costs of room and board expensive. It was to the advantage of the student to stay near home.

2. As these new schools arose, competition among them became serious and damaging to the training offered. The original term of lectures was seven to nine months a year for two years, including clinical and bedside training. Within a few years this declined to four or five months. Admission requirements also declined with competency in Latin, mathematics, and the natural sciences no longer required. Whitfield J. Bell, Jr., in his 1960 article on the early years of the Yale School of Medicine, commented on the quality of admitted medical students in 1850-51; he noted that, while 80% of divinity students had bachelor's degrees, as did 65% of law students, only 26% of medical students entered with that level of competency.[1]

3. Financial gain for the physicians who were the faculty of these schools was a major incentive for them. Tuition for admission to the school and the salary as professor were appealing attractions for local physicians.

4. There was a certain prestige to being a professor in a medical school, not unknown in any era. Also, this prestige had an obvious and positive influence on enlarging a private practice.

5. Rural communities in the expanding nation could look with pride on the existence of a medical school in their town, placing them nearly on the level with the cities and their colleges.

6. For many physicians the local medical school also offered an alternative to having apprentices in the office taking up time and space that could be better - and more profitably - used seeing patients.

All in all, then, the nineteenth century saw an amazing growth in medical schools that accepted poorly educated students, offered minimal education and training, were highly competitive for a limited number of students, and played upon the worst motives of the doctors who founded them. A solution to the problem of a medical education sadly lacking in proper learning opportunities and clinical training was offered at some schools. The same faculty that taught the regular term also offered a 'private school' that students could attend off-season for a fee. The classes were small and the instruction more personal. For those who could afford it, this added study offered a distinct advantage.

In his article on the early years of the Medical Institution of Yale College noted above, Bell described the plight of the school. The small faculty of six physicians had local reputations only, and, at one time three of them were brothers-in-law. Competition with the proprietary schools resulted in decreasing enrollments, and the reputation of the school was that of a training school for Connecticut doctors. Bell wrote,

> [T]he Medical Institution faced the competition from new schools throughout the country which offered degrees for less money, time, and study, and the institutions in New York and Boston which provided opportunities for laboratory work and hospital visitation that New Haven could not hope to equal. Yale was thus in the awkward position of being unable, because of its university connection, to compete with the poor schools and unable, because of New Haven's limited clinical facilities, to compete with the best.[2]

This, then, was the sad state of American medical education in much of that nineteenth century. The impact of this situation on the reputation of the profession and the quality of the skills of its physicians was negative at best, disastrous for patients at worst. Washington Hooker, a prominent physician in Connecticut in the middle years of the nineteenth century, noted in his Report of the Committee on Medical Education to the 1851 meeting of the American Medical Association,

> The national literature of our profession is impressed with the great fact that uneducated predominates very largely over educated talent among medical men in this country. While there is no lack of energy or fruitfulness, there is a great want of chasteness of style and correctness of reasoning, There is an abundance of loose observation, and careless inferences, and ingenious but useless theorizing; for untrained minds are apt to speculate, and to be fond of mere illustration and analogy in place of argument.[3]

The Heroic Age

The first half of the nineteenth century is known as the Heroic Age in medicine. This label derives from the vigorous means employed to treat diseases - usually fevers - in that time. From our contemporary viewpoint by far and away the most alarming was the practice of bloodletting, using a lancet to open a vein and draw off blood, often a pint at a time. The major exponent of this treatment method was Benjamin Rush, a physician who was considered in his day the leading physician in America. Rush received his M.D. in 1769 from Edinburgh where he idolized his teacher, William Cullen. In Rush's autobiography, *Travels Through Life,* he wrote, "The two years I spent in Edinburgh I consider as the most important in their influence upon my character and conduct of any period of my life."[4] The System that Cullen proposed placed the cause of disease in abnormalities in the functions of small blood vessels that he called "spasms." Treatments consisted of alterations in diet, cold baths, purging and bloodletting. Rush, deciding that fevers were caused by severe spasms only in the arteries, settled on bloodletting as *the* treatment for most diseases, particularly for fevers.

Recalling that the diagnoses of most diseases were made by listening to the history of the patient, taking the pulse, and looking at the urine, it is not surprising that treatments that produced changes evident to the observers - patient, family, and doctor - were considered successful. Thus bloodletting that produced pallor, cool skin, and an altered pulse was obviously effective. Nathan G. Goodman, in his 1934 biography of Rush, wrote,

> In his theory of the proximate cause of fever, Rush explained that fever is caused directly by the morbid and excessive action of the blood vessels,...In defending bloodletting, Rush pointed out that the blood is the most powerful stimulus acting upon the vessels and fibre, and, by withdrawing a part of it, the principal cause of the fever is diminished in its potency.[5]

To this amazing treatment was added severe purging, leeches, drugs that caused vomiting, and opium for pain. Rush offers an excellent example of a theoretical medical System where both the causes of diseases and appropriate treatments are essentially invented in the mind of the doctor with minimal understanding of the physiological or pathological processes determining the illness. As John Harley Warner pointed out in his 1997 study of therapeutics in these years,

> Heroic depletive practices gave clear evidence that they worked....[W]hen a patient with a hard, fast pulse, high temperature, and delirium became calmer - physiologically lower - after a large volume of blood had been let, the treatment's effect was undeniable. Sleep promoted by opiates further testified to the ability of the physician to alter his patient's physiology at will. Confirmation of the treatment's efficacy was generally rapid,...[6]

The combination of immediate and obvious response also testified to the skill of the physician and established the validity of the method. Of course, in that time there were little, if any, laboratory studies available; invention was the master of medicine.

Rush, appointed professor of chemistry at Philadelphia in 1769 at twenty-three, was an outstanding physician in his day: attractive, intelligent, careful, and forceful, he became a major figure in American medicine. Since so many newly educated physicians were trained at Philadelphia, bloodletting and purging became major treatments for almost all diseases.

In our day Rush is associated only with the horrors implicit in bleeding patients, removing large quantities of blood from ill persons. However, there are other aspects to his professional life that are impressive. He was one of the first American physicians to be interested in the care of the seriously mentally ill, whom he referred to as the 'insane' and 'madmen.' Rush has been called America's first psychiatrist. He succeeded in establishing an asylum for psychiatric patients, treating some, of course, by bloodletting and others by spinning them in a centrifuge-like chair to send more blood to the brain. Rush also advocated a cleaner city with wider streets, more care in attending to garbage and other wastes, decreasing the number of medical nostrums, and making diagnostic categories simpler and easier to understand. He was a remarkable man.

After his death in 1813, his System of diagnosis and treatment prevailed for decades. In those years an accepted aspect of medical practice was the treatment of symptoms. Specific diagnoses of diseases were uncommon with obvious exceptions such as smallpox, scarlet fever, cholera, and consumption. The main purpose of the doctor was to treat symptoms, and in ways that made treatment results obvious. Another determinative factor in American medicine in the first two-thirds of the nineteenth century was the concept of specificity, the conviction that there were specific facts about a patient and that patient's environment that sharply defined therapy because they also defined symptoms. Personality traits such as temperament and bodily constitution, the climate where one lived, the work one did, and one's family makeup - all these were to be considered in determining treatment. The doctor did not treat a disease, he treated a patient. Of course, one of the outstanding factors was race, clearly separating treatment options.

The severity of the depletive therapies of bloodletting and purging also provided the basis for the rapid development and proliferation of alternatives to treatment by regular physicians. Coincident with the poor training physicians received and the frightening therapies they offered was this search for other methods of treatment. This was supported, in turn, by the deterioration in medical education described above. Central to understanding these changes was a radical shift in the thinking and acting of American voters in response to a new political and social vision of the nation based upon the expanding western frontier. Before proceeding further with my medical historical narrative we need some background information on what is almost a second American Revolution.

The Era of Jacksonian Democracy

Andrew Jackson was elected President of the United States in 1828 and served two terms as the seventh President. An army general - and a popular hero - in the War of 1812, his election was a turning point in American political history. In the decades preceding his election there were questions raised by elected officials concerning the wisdom and the morality of democracy. Most of the men who governed were from the eastern seaboard, were well educated, and came from the higher levels of society. There were concerns about the abilities of the average man to perform the tasks and bear the serious responsibilities of government. Into this setting came a powerful actor.

Jackson was born in humble circumstances. The first President from west of Appalachia, he had experience with frontier life and identified himself as a member of the populace. He was close to the mass of people, made a powerful appeal to them, and had a very strong and persistent commitment to democratic processes, based upon his sense of the importance of everyman in government. He was essentially elected as the candidate of the people, not of a political party. There was almost a reversal in understanding the functions of government. Doubts about the extent of power exerted by government over the daily lives of the people became an issue. Regulations and restrictions on personal and business ventures were criticized and rejected in the name of equal opportunities for all.

Jackson's two terms of office firmly determined the two-party system in American politics. Another result of his election was the demonstration of the westward movement of America and the opening of what seemed to be an endless frontier for expansion: for development of individuals, economic possibilities, and unlicensed practices of any type.

A New Age in Medicine

In colonial America, even before the founding of medical schools, quackery was ever-present, and reports in the press and in public statements pointed out the very obvious abuses foisted on the people by untrained persons interested only in making money by treating a gullible and uneducated public. Efforts were made to correct this, and in 1760 the first regulatory law was passed for New York City that required an examination of all students seeking to practice medicine. By 1830 thirteen states had passed similar laws for licensing physicians. Instrumental in these legislative efforts were physicians who had organized both state and local (or county) medical societies, the first organized in Boston in 1735. Others followed and worked with state legislatures to bring some order into stabilizing rules for practicing medicine.

In response to the new democratic concepts that became so powerful in the 1830s however, these licensing laws were repealed, and by 1850 only two states and Washington, D.C. still had them. The repeal of these laws cleared the way for rampant quackery provided by physicians and anyone else calling himself a doctor or a healer. Since even the earlier laws usually did not require an examination, only proof that the applicant have a degree, attendance at a proprietary school that offered minimal education and no training paved the way to widespread and harmful quackery. It also created the phenomenon of the 'diploma mill.' If all that was required to practice medicine was a degree, then enterprising men found ways to offer a degree by mail for a fee. The result of this new system was a profusion of 'doctors' with no medical education. It would require a major effort by properly trained physicians acting through their medical societies and with the legislatures to finally overcome this new barrier to proper medical care.

Another result of the rapid spread of Jacksonian democratic beliefs was the appearance on the American scene of herbalists and other persons offering cures for most ailments. Several factors were important in the emergence of this new phenomenon.

1. With the spread of proprietary medical colleges offering degrees after very inadequate education, and often absent training, the number of persons labeled 'doctor' increased rapidly. Their skills were minimal and often extremely hazardous since they knew so little. Soon, the mere word, doctor, was enough to send patients in search of other healers.

2. Growing dismay in the public eye with heroic medical practices of orthodox practitioners - especially bloodletting and purging with

poisons such as mercury - opened the field to those who offered milder cures with vegetable and herbal concoctions that did not insult the body beyond its limits of endurance. By the middle of the nineteenth century there was widespread suspicion, anger, and antagonism directed at physicians because of their treatment regimens. As might be anticipated, this antagonism caused physicians to close ranks and defend themselves rather that becoming open to what was happening. Bloodletting became a symbol of the profession. Empirics - those who used treatments because they worked - were ridiculed by physicians.

3. There appeared, in small towns in particular, traveling doctors who offered their services as specialists, supposedly superior to local practitioners trained as apprentices. Advertising their special talents and abilities in the local newspaper, and claiming to be highly trained, they were usually quacks passing through and seeking gullible patients.

4. The democratic impulse also discredited doctors as persons who advertised themselves in ways that made them seem superior. Doctors also struggled during these middle years of the century to establish settled fees for their work that seemed excessive to the public. Those who offered less painful treatments and lower prices were, therefore, sought out by the sick and disabled. There was a distrust rampant in the country that supported the idea that, not only could we perhaps treat ourselves by advertised remedies, but that we could be treated by others like us who might be able to help.

These various factors opened the door to an astounding array of irregular doctors and healers in the nineteenth century. These irregulars, referred to as quacks by trained physicians, became an epidemic. Washington Hooker wrote in 1849 that,

> Quackery has, at length, come to be so monstrous an evil, that there will be great difficulty in removing it. The credulity of the public is so great and so extensive, that the plainest and strongest facts, brought out even in multitudinous array, are almost powerless before it.[7]

These same elements were important, of course, in the repeal of licensing laws. Four sectarian healers offer us a glimpse into this remarkable world.

1. Elisha Perkins began his practice of medicine in 1759 in Norwich, Connecticut. In those times there was interest in the discoveries of the wonders of electricity illustrated so clearly by Benjamin Franklin. Perkins, in 1795, apparently reasoning that rheumatic pains were

caused by an excess of electricity in muscles and joints, experimented with drawing a knife blade over the painful part, with amazing success. He made metallic tractors, had the process patented, and proceeded to sell them at a nice profit. He died in the yellow fever epidemic of 1799, but his son went on to a very profitable career in England and in Denmark. Joseph F. Kett, in his 1968 book, *The Formation of The American Medical Profession,* wrote,

> Elisha Perkins himself was a queer amalgam of educated physician and charlatan, genuinely believing he had made a major scientific discovery but willing to distort its nature for profit....Perkinism never became a medical sect; it lacked a coherent medical theory applicable to all ailments....In the thirties and forties regulatory laws were confronted and destroyed by a new type of medical creed.[8]

This new medical creed was Thomsonianism.

2. Samuel Thomson was born in New Hampshire in 1769, the son of a Baptist farmer. He developed an enduring interest in plants, learning their names and medical uses from a female herbal practitioner. By the time he was in his twenties he had decided to become a healer and he developed a system of treatment based upon his understanding of the construction of all animal bodies as comprised of the Hippocratic-like elements of fire, air, water, and earth. Based on Galen-like reasoning, he advised the use of steam baths, emetics and purgatives not unlike his contemporary regular physicians. His practice extended steadily and he soon had an impressive reputation as a healer. His therapeutic system was basically botanical, not significantly different from colonial herbal healers.

Thomson received a patent for his system which was sold for twenty dollars to people who would then form Friendly Botanical Societies to learn and to teach the fundamentals of his system. It was a firm belief that only some people had a power to heal others, and that a medical education would not supply the power if it was not already there. This System became very popular and various sources estimate that several million persons across the country preferred herbal therapy to orthodox medical treatment. There was very strong support of Thomsonianism from the clergy who found this new system to be one that pointed toward the gradual perfectionism of the human race. In these years of the second Great Awakening in America, this new way of healing that championed the abilities of average people to heal was acclaimed as a welcome reform in morality as well as in health. Other positive and appealing aspects of Thomsonianism were moderation in diet, and abstinence from alcohol and tobacco.

Two fundamental commitments of the Thomsonians were to support democracy and the power of the people, and oppose aristocratic and regulatory systems, especially the elite medical profession that was struggling unsuccessfully across the nation to hold, however inadequately, to its position of authority and competence. In the era of Jacksonian Democracy the Thomsonians found widespread support. John S. Haller, Jr., in his 1999 study of alternative medicine commented that

> What began as a protest against the heroic practices of regular medicine turned into a mass movement that swept through the back roads of rural and small-town America. The particular strength of Thomson's system was its democratic appeal.[9]

Another powerful factor in the popularity of this sect was its complete acceptance of women as healers and as participants in the structure of the herbal societies. Thomsonians saw themselves as reformers in the most profound sense, allying their cause to that of Martin Luther and others as they attempted to turn the face of America to pure democracy. Kett, in commenting on the contribution of Thomson, wrote,

> [W]ith the rise of perfectionism disease became intolerable. It seemed impossible that a benevolent God would ruthlessly consign the greater portion of mankind to protracted pain. Thomson's contribution lay in harnessing this perfectionist ardor to the realities of a still rural society where a great deal of medical practice was inevitably domestic. For all its crudity, Thomsonianism was, in a way, scientific.[10]

3. The Eclectics developed as a sect of botanic practitioners that stood in opposition to both allopathic - regular or orthodox - doctors and Thomsonians. Instrumental in its inception was Wooster Beach (1794-1868), a graduate of New York's College of Physicians and Surgeons. After a few years of practice, in response to his distaste for heroic chemical therapy, he developed his own system of treatments based upon the gentle use of vegetable remedies. Beach was well instructed in botanical literature and sought kinder treatments for his patients. He opened a school in 1825, expanded it in 1829, and the following year it was named the Reformed Medical College of the City of New York. The use of the word, reformed, is a signal of its import for the remarkable democratic era just beginning.

Beach published his popular three-volume textbook on medical practice in 1833 that presented his views on the nature of reform needed in medicine to counter the ancient foundations of current practice that relied on violent physical and chemical therapies. Haller offered a review of eclectic principles:

> In general, the eclectics favored the natural curative processes of the organism through the use of noninjurious medication; demanded freedom of thought and investigation; supported the development of the vegetable materia medica as the safest method of treating disease; supported the inductive method of investigation; advocated simplicity in prescribing; determined the value of a drug through treatment of the sick patient rather than through laboratory experimentation; and condemned the extremes of over drugging and therapeutic nihilism.[11]

Unable to receive a charter in New York, a western affiliate was opened at the invitation of Worthington College in Ohio in 1830. In 1845 several schools joined forces and received a charter from the State of Ohio to become the Eclectic Medical Institute of Cincinnati. This school became the Eclectic Medical College in 1910, finally closing its doors in 1939 in response to new and profound changes in medical education in the United States that I will present later.

4. Homeopathy (from the Greek, *homios,* like) is a method of medical practice based upon the idea that diseases can be cured - or at least treated - by very small doses of drugs that, given in large amounts to a healthy person, cause the same symptoms as the disease. Samuel Christian Friedrich Hahnemann (1755-1843) was a German physician who developed and taught this doctrine after his studies of the effects of cinchona bark on himself that produced fever, thus explaining its therapeutic value in treating malaria. Hahnemann published his textbook in 1810, a work that would become a standard text in America. Hahnemann also had a spiritual component to his thought that was attractive to the times.

Imported into the United States in the 1830s and 1840s, homeopathy ("like cures like") became increasingly popular, especially among the large immigrant populations in the Northeast. By the 1870s it was the leading sect in America: by 1900 there was one homeopathic physician for every ten regular doctors. Obviously this sect was an overwhelming threat to those physicians still practicing heroic medicine. Martin Kaufman, commenting on the success of this sect, wrote,

> Many orthodox physicians recognized this and cast aside the lancet and calomel in favor of the infinitesimal doses of homeopathy. It seemed evident that aside from any benefits that might be wrought by homeopathic treatment, the orthodox physicians were eliminating those patients who

were too ill to endure heroic practices while the homeopaths were saving patients through supportive treatment.[12]

A major positive result of the homeopathic process was a very careful taking of the history of the patient and close attention to personal details in that history that might be attended to by a thoughtful and caring physician.   This new arrival on the American scene, Homeopathy, will be discussed further in my study of William Henry Holcombe.

In the years just preceding the Civil War, American medicine was falling apart.   There were too many medical schools providing extremely inadequate education; hospitals for proper bedside clinical training were hard to find, and that training was not required; there were too many doctors attracted to the profession by the ease of becoming one; efforts at educational reform by some of the schools associated with universities were failing;   licensing by examination was almost nonexistent; attempts to organize the medical profession were proceeding haltingly.   The profession was caught in a dilemma: there was a growing interest in the traditional sciences of chemistry and physics and the new and exciting sciences of physiology and pathology that were pointing to the definition of specific diseases by experimental and laboratory methodologies; there was also counterbalancing intense loyalty to the history of the profession and its defining methods of treating symptoms by bleeding and purging.

There was change in the air, though.   The habit of some American doctors to go abroad to continue their studies had persisted and their destinations became France and Germany where new theories and practices were evolving at an exciting rate.   Most doctors who went abroad in the 1820s to the 1840s were from the Northeast, creating a certain elitism in the profession with expected consequences in the responses of those who stayed at home.   Change was in the offing, however, and in succeeding years American physicians by the thousands went to Europe to be a part of the excitement of the new learning, the European Experience.

The European Experience
Paris

The French Revolution that erupted in 1789 caused remarkable changes in medical education and practice in France.   The preceding era of the Enlightenment had fostered the construction of hospitals and some attention to public health, but the status of education and the care of patients were very poor. Death rates in the leading Paris hospital were more than twice those in London hospitals. The standard distinctions between physicians and surgeons were carefully preserved, and theory was the basis for understanding the symptoms of disease and controlling treatments.

In 1794 the Convention received a report on the status of medical care in France prepared by a chemist, Antoine Fourcroy, and a physician, François Chaussier, that became the basis for a 'revolutionary' law that laid the foundation for a new center of medical education for Europe and America - Paris. The Revolution, with its powerful egalitarian influences, hoped to dismantle hospitals that were filthy, overcrowded, and a hazard to the public. They, along with traditional elite doctors, would be replaced by a new system of home care providers. This anti-establishment hope bears some close resemblance to the sectarian moves in America that supported herbalism, homeopathy, and other outlying treatment methods that were so opposed to traditional medicine. The expanding wars in Europe with the demand for military surgeons pressed for a reform, not only of medical education, but of other scientific schools for which competitive examinations were required. In a brief time there was a massive change in medical education.

Three medical schools were formed in France with uniform requirements for educational standards, faculty qualifications, and licensing. A major part of the new law of 1794 was the establishment of medicine and surgery as equal partners of the newly emerging science of medicine. Of course, the demand for military surgeons played a distinct role in this ruling, but it also had important conceptual meanings for education. W.F. Bynum, in his 1994 book, *Science and the Practice of Medicine in the Nineteenth Century,* noted that the law equalized physicians and surgeons in the hospital. In addition,

> It had even more important consequences for medical thought, for it taught generations of students to conceptualize disease as surgeons would: in terms of anatomic structures, the solid parts, local lesions. This systematic integration created the ambience for the emphasis on pathology, physical diagnosis, and clinicopathological correlation, which are the hallmarks of hospital medicine.[13]

In a very short period of time the medical school in Paris became the gem of the new medical educational system.

The Paris School, fabled as it was, - and is - had an amazing number of talented and imaginative teachers. Lawrence Brockliss and Colin

Jones wrote, in their 1997 text, *The Medical World of Early Modern France,* that

> The Founder of the Paris School is usually held to be Marie-François-Xavier Bichat (1771-1802) who, paradoxically, was neither a public professor nor an academically trained physician....His legacy lay in his passionate commitment to careful and endlessly repeated dissections. Bichat turned French anatomy into a science rather than a piece of casual theatre....[14]

According to William Osler, Bichat's textbook, *Anatomie Generale,* "laid the foundation of the positive or modern method of the study of medicine, in which theory and reasoning were replaced by observation and analysis."[15]One can see why Paris began to draw students to it from Britain, Germany, and America. John Harley Warner opened his 1998 book, *Against the Spirit of System* with this note:

> What has come to be called the Paris Clinical School is broadly identified with a distinctive complex of institutional arrangements, clinical techniques and teaching practices, modes of organizing knowledge, and structures of medical perception that characterized Paris medicine between 1794 and the mid-nineteenth century....Paris became a Mecca for foreign medical students and practitioners....The knowledge, techniques, and ideals these travelers brought back were leading ingredients in the transformation of American medicine before the Civil War, so much so that historians have called the antebellum era the "French period" in American medicine.[16]

There were several other aspects of the new system that led to changes that would persist to our times. Teachers in the new schools and hospitals were salaried, permitting them to devote their energies to teaching and to research. Also, positions were created for internships and externships that would open the door to an academic future for outstanding students. Formal examinations were required for graduation and a license to practice.

From the beginning of the student's education, bedside teaching was central. Careful observation of patients would lead to understanding the course that a disease takes; analysis of physical examinations of a large number of patients would lead to classifications that would provide a structure for evaluation of therapies; finally, availability of human bodies, both for anatomical study and for pathological investigation at autopsy, completed the setting for a new and very attractive education and training to become a competent doctor.

There were a number of physicians in what would be known as the Paris School who were outstanding attractions to students and to other physicians. J. N. Corvisart (1755-1821) was a professor of medicine at the Paris medical school. He translated a brief 1761 work, *Inventum novum,* by Leopold Auenbrugger on percussion of the chest. This Viennese physician learned the technique of tapping with his fingers when he was required to determine the level between fluid and air in the wine casks in the cellar of his father's inn. Corvisart added this technique to his teaching, further emphasizing the importance of the triangular relationships among the history of the patient, the physical examination, and the findings at autopsy.

One of the greatest physicians in Paris was R.T.H. Laennec (1781-1826), discoverer of the stethoscope in 1816 during his examination of an obese woman whose breath and heart sounds were inaudible. Rolling a piece of paper into a tube, he was able to hear both heart and breath sounds. Within a few years the stethoscope became a symbol of the profession and has remained so. Laennec became a prominent teacher, documenting his findings with care; his experiences led him, as it did so many others, to a position of therapeutic nihilism: the treatments offered by doctors had little curative effect on major diseases of heart and lungs.

Pierre-Charles-Alexandre Louis was one of the Paris School teachers who followed on the heels of Bichat. A pupil of Auguste-François Chomel, Louis spent some six years studying diseases by gathering facts based upon anatomical dissection and correlation with physical findings of patients. Historically, Louis, through a method of patient-treatment analysis called the Numerical Method, became the symbol of a complete transformation in both clinical and therapeutic thinking in medicine; thus, his fame and his appeal in the 1830s. Louis understood clinical medicine to be an observational science: careful analysis of the symptoms of a patient, the treatments given, and the results of those treatments either by recovery of the patient or at the autopsy table. In his time the sciences of physiology, biochemistry, microscopy, and cellular biology were in their infancy, if even born yet. Louis stressed the importance of immaculate data collection and its analysis mathematically. One could say that the emphasis of Louis was to teach students to attend to their senses: what they saw, touched, smelled and heard was what would establish a diagnosis and evaluate a therapy. William Osler found the concerted efforts during this period of study by Louis to be unique in medical history. The Numerical Method, he wrote, so simple, so self-evident, we owe largely to Louis, in whose hands it proved an invaluable instrument of research. He [Louis] remarks in one place that the edifice of medicine reposes entirely upon facts, and that truth cannot be elicited but from those which have been well and completely observed.[17]

One of the crucial studies of Louis was on the efficacy of bloodletting in the treatment of pneumonia, a standard practice in America. His evidence of the uselessness of this heroic therapy was instrumental in the practice finally dying out. From an historical perspective, in keeping with one of the hypotheses of this study, we can see the ease of finding in the history of medicine opposing and co-existing theories firmly believed and convincingly argued. At the very moment when the Numerical Method was prominent, there were those who saw it as a static understanding of disease. One of the most important contributions of the Method was the documentation of diseases as specific entities; the demonstrable pathological findings, not the symptoms, determined the diagnosis. But there were physicians and teachers who were convinced that there were physiological processes that, when interrupted or lost, caused the symptoms that led to the diagnosis of the patient. To these physicians there was an inflexibility in understanding diseases only from studies of dead bodies. Living processes determine our wellness and our sickness.

It was not long before students from all over came to Paris to study. The attractions of the hospitals were spectacular: foreign students were welcome and could attend lectures and clinics as they desired; human anatomy studies were readily available and private teachers were easily found; the most prominent physicians of the leading medical school in the world were right there in the theatre, the clinic, the hospital ward. Americans were welcomed into the various social and medical clubs in Paris, and a number of Americans stayed for several years, serving as *internes* or *externes* to professors at the Paris School. But there was another side to Paris that was of concern particularly to Americans: they were appalled at what they took to be the moral laxness of Parisians, the street and cafe life. Many Americans came from a strong Puritanical family background and were distressed by what they saw, not only on the streets, but in the hospital. There seemed to be a certain disinterest in the treatment of patients, with physicians showing a deeper concern for matching symptoms with autopsy findings than providing care and comfort for the sick. Public sanitation was also noted to be in poor repair and both the streets and the hospitals were dirty and unattractive to men and women from the more sparsely settled American shores.

The American experience in Paris was, on the whole, a good one. Quick acceptance into the hospital system, free access to lectures and clinics, and the new realization of an empirical approach to medicine based upon observation, not invention - all these were extremely attractive to Americans. Central to this experience was bedside teaching, the opportunity to learn from the histories and the physical examinations of readily available patients the techniques of accurate diagnosis that could then be confirmed at surgery or autopsy. This experience would be invaluable upon returning to the United States and entering into competition with the myriad of doctors, so many of whom were graduates of inadequate proprietary schools. Warner, commenting in his discussion of why Americans chose Paris rather than London, wrote,

> Study in Paris, then, represented a catalyst for transforming the inexperienced graduate into a seasoned practitioner, with all the material and emotional rewards anticipated from such a change. Experience at the bedside, moreover, gave the physician self-assurance and poise that generated confidence in patients,...[18]

There were several aspects of hospital practice in Paris that distressed Americans, making their praise of the Paris School somewhat ambiguous on their return. Americans found the French lack of concern for the *care* of patients abhorrent. Disinterest in the outcome of an illness- except in the pathological findings - and a serious disregard for the modesty of women patients were distressing. There seemed to be a relationship between the observed immorality apparent in Parisian street life and the lack of moral principles Americans detected in their instructors' dealings with patients. There was a harshness in Paris hospital practice that dismayed Americans and made them assess very carefully how they would interpret their experiences in Paris for their future patients. In the era of Jacksonian democracy, widespread alternative healing sects, and a dislike for foreign influences, devotees of the Paris School, upon their return home, were very cautious in their presentation of the importance of their training there. Confident in the superior clinical training they had received, they were also aware of the impersonal attitude that many of their Parisian teachers held toward their patients. It was a balancing act to hold in creative positions both the empiricism of Parisian medicine that undercut most theories supporting therapeutic intervention, and the American commitment to treating the sick.

In January 1855 the dean of the faculty of the School of Paris discontinued private teaching of students by the *internes*. This was an important decision; overcrowding in lecture halls and in clinics made private instruction central to the Paris experience, and its loss began the decline of Paris as the center for medical training. This was not immediate, of course, but it did signal the beginning of a very important shift of students to the rising stars of Vienna and Berlin. Laboratory experience in Paris in physiology, pathology, and pharmacology under the tutelage of François Magendie (1783-1855) and his star pupil Claude Bernard (1813-1878) was superb, but lacked the strong support of the medical school that was so important to the growth of German biological sciences. There was a combination of events that led to the decline, in American eyes, of the Paris School for medical education: loss of private instruction and crowded lecture halls, the observed callousness of physicians for care of patients, the inevitable deaths of leading teachers, and the insecure position of laboratory sciences in that education. However, by the middle years of the nineteenth century medical training in Europe had become a necessity: it was crucial for those Americans seeking an excellent education; it was a brief but delightful vacation for some; for others it was a nice addition to one's *curriculum vitae*. Those going to Europe sought another setting where their educational needs could be met with assurance.

The European Experience
Vienna and Germany

By the 1850s Vienna became a central locus for medical training. The hospital facilities were extensive and accessible to foreigners, private instruction was readily available, and the laboratory sciences were developing rapidly. American students found the same unattractive clinical attributes of physicians in Vienna and in German university medical schools that they criticized in Paris: callousness, disinterest in therapy, and a stress on accurate diagnosis confirmed at autopsy.

But there was a new horizon appearing in medical science. Laboratory investigation in Germany was often an integral part of a scientific Institute that was itself part of a university whose investigators were full-time professors able to do their work without concerns for maintaining a private practice. Students worked closely with their professors, side-by-side, in their laboratories. The microscope was now an affordable instrument and optically well-made; this transformed both biological investigation and the practice of medicine. The cell became the new focus for the study of diseases. Laboratory investigation fascinated this new generation of doctors and opened opportunities for them to choose between two possible careers: to become a physician-clinician or a physician-scientist. Attractive as the new laboratory sciences were, physicians were aware of contrary opinions about science in the minds of the public. Bynum noted several concerns of these scientists:

> They were conscious...of a potential public distrust or even fear of too much fondness for science among those entrusted with their health, and with access to their bodies....[D]octors in the 1830s would have been aware of public loathing of anatomical dissection, of the poor's fear of hospitals as places where they might be experimented upon (or treatment withheld in the interests of following the "natural history" of the disease),...[19]

However, there would be no turning back. The cellular basis for living organisms in both normal and diseased conditions could not be denied. Unfortunately, the new biological sciences held out expectations and hopes for therapy that would not be realized for another century.

New Visions, New Times

The Civil War brought into painfully sharp view the abject condition of the training of American physicians that I have described above. Their care of soldiers was woefully inadequate: anatomical knowledge was poor, the use of the stethoscope was unknown, examination of eye and ear by instruments was a rarity, and pharmacology was not part of their armamentarium. Surgical skills for many medical officers were learned when they first treated gunshot wounds. Disease and poor medical care caused a higher death rate than combat.

Following the war, the last third of the nineteenth century was a time of phenomenal changes in medicine. The war had stimulated rapid growth in industries and in the new technologies that accompanied them. There was a profusion of new knowledge, an information explosion that effected many aspects of professional and business life. A crucial part of this growth was the renewal of public education. Of course, Horace Mann (1796-1859), appointed in 1837 to be the secretary of the first state board of education in Massachusetts, was the tireless proponent of a system that would have its snowball effects felt in the universities that were beginning to form. The university became the home of research in the new sciences. Educational methods were rethought in both the humanities and in the sciences. Physicians returning home from studies in Paris and in Germany found positions as professors where they could continue their laboratory investigations. The improvements in public education raised the standards of undergraduate training that would be felt in some of the medical schools. Although proprietary schools still prospered, there was a developing interest in universities for including medical schools in their structure. The relationships between medicine and science were recognized and expanded, bringing into existence the great schools that would make American medical schools the model for the world.

Kenneth M. Ludmerer, in his comprehensive 1985 study of this period, *Learning to Heal,* summarized these events and wrote that,

> in the 1870s and 1880s the underlying developments that would later make possible the rapid and dramatic improvements in medical education in the Progressive Era were already underway. Medical knowledge was rapidly increasing, and mastery thereof was becoming more and more important to the practice of good medicine. A cadre of teachers was arising, intent on transmitting scientific medicine to their students. The university was developing, preparing to provide a home for modern medical education. And the supply of students educationally qualified to begin the rigorous study of medicine was becoming much larger.[20]

Partakers in these eventful times and contributors to the phenomenal advances in medicine that occurred in the century between the years 1830 and 1920 were some notable American physicians. I have chosen a representative group that will demonstrate various aspects of our personalities that can make a difference in our world and the work we do in it: our individuality, inventiveness, compassion, insights into human nature, and our commitment to change. These women and men offer us examples of intellectual effort and personal behavior that illustrate the possibilities for altering the human condition. Again, I would stress the central concern of this study: at the very moment that history is moving in one direction, thoughtful and responsible persons are seeking a change in direction. Behind historical events are persons who work toward the fulfillment of expectations, be they good or bad for our human condition. There are those of us who see the evils perpetrated in our world and make the decision to work for changes that will alleviate suffering, improve health, protect the helpless, comfort the afflicted. This study looks at some of these persons who were physicians in the renaissance years of the nineteenth and early twentieth centuries.

[1]Bell, Jr., Whitfield J., "The Medical Institution of Yale College, 1810-1885," *Yale Journal of Biology and Medicine,* (33), December 1960, 174.

[2]Bell, Ibid., 174.

[3]Hooker, Worthington, "Report of the Committee on Medical Education," extracted from *The Transactions of the American Medical Association,* Philadelphia, T.K. and P.G. Collins, 1851, 19.

[4]Rush, Benjamin, *The Autobiography of Benjamin Rush,* edited by George W. Corner, Princeton, Princeton University Press, 1948, 43.

[5]Goodman, Nathan G., *Benjamin Rush: Physician and Citizen,* Philadelphia, University of Pennsylvania Press, 1934, 248.

[6]Warner, John Harley, *The Therapeutic Perspective,* Princeton, Princeton University Press, 1997, 92.

[7]Hooker, Worthington, *Physician and Patient,* New York, Baker and Scribner, 1849, 90-91.

[8]Kett, Joseph F., *The Formation of the American Medical Profession,* New Haven, Yale University Press, 1968, 99-100.

[9]Haller, Jr., John S., *A Profile in Alternative Medicine,* Kent, Ohio, The Kent University Press, 1999, 13.

[10]Kett, *op. cit.,* 131.

[11]Haller, *op. cit.,* 19.

[12]Kaufman, Martin, *American Medical Education: The Formative Years,1765-1910,* Westport, Ct., Greenwood Press,71.

[13]Bynum, W.F., *Science and the Practice of Medicine in the Nineteenth Century,* Cambridge, Cambridge University Press, 1994, 28.

[14]Brockliss, Lawrence, and Jones, Colin, *The Medical World of Early Modern France,* Oxford, Clarendon Press, 1997, 826.

[15]Osler, William, "The Influence of Louis on American Medicine," *An Alabama Student and Other Biographical Essays,* London, Oxford University Press, 1908, 189.

[16]Warner, John Harley, *Against the Spirit of System,* Princeton, Princeton University Press, 1998, 3.

[17]Osler, *op. cit.,* 193.

[18]Warner, *Against the Spirit...,* *op. cit.,* 42.

[19]Bynum, *op. cit.,* 93.

[20]Ludmerer, Kenneth M., *Learning to Heal,* New York, Basic Books, 1985, 46.

Chapter 3

Jacob Bigelow, 1787-1879

To begin our biographical study of physicians who effected a renaissance - a new birth - in American medicine I chose Jacob Bigelow, a Boston physician who was, in himself, somewhat of a Renaissance man. In the very era of the disintegration of medical education and practice, and the eruption of quackery and sectarian therapies, Bigelow is the stellar example of the thoughtful and caring doctor whose life is informed by observation and study.

Student Years

Jacob Bigelow was born in Sudbury, Massachusetts, the part of Watertown that is now called Waltham. He was the second son of a clergyman who divided his time between his 30-40 acre farm and the parish he served for forty years. The family was poor, but still the expectation was that Bigelow would attend Harvard College, as had his father. Bigelow attended public school five or six months a year, as permitted by the duties of harvesting and planting. His father, perhaps aware either of the dawning of industrialism or the decline in the status of the clergy, discouraged his son from reading the classics; in fact, he locked up his Latin and Greek texts, recommending arithmetic and writing as suitable for the times. Bigelow did manage to find a Latin Grammar that he studied in the woods. In the future he would be proficient in writing in Latin, much to the surprise of some of his critics. At the age of thirteen Bigelow was sent to Weston with some other boys to live with a Reverend Samuel Kendall, a minister who taught young boys to 'fit them out' for college. It was assumed that the sons of alumni would follow their fathers.

Bigelow was a student at Harvard at a time of serious instability in administration, teaching, and finances. The school had not yet recovered from the dislocations of the Revolutionary War, the faculty was limited in number and abilities, and the physical facilities were quite insufficient. However, Bigelow did well as a student, joined all the clubs and societies, and graduated Phi Beta Kappa in 1806 at the age of nineteen. He was a good student and he went on to receive his master's degree; at commencement - as a mark of his scholarship - he was offered the opportunity to give the English Oration, an honor he declined, concerned as he was about the quality of his public speaking skills.

Choosing a Career

For college graduates in those years three careers - the three learned professions - were the only options: law, clergy, and medicine. Only the first was considered both honorable and assuring of the provision of a decent and reliable living. The status of the clergy in New England had declined considerably in the years after the War, only about half of the sons of ministers following in their fathers' footsteps. As we noted earlier, the work of doctors as purgers, bleeders, and pushers of pills probably held little attraction for Bigelow. Also, Bigelow had decided that, after his childhood experiences, country life was not for him. In his senior year at Harvard, Dr. John Warren, the eldest in a distinguished line of Boston physicians, gave a series of lectures on anatomy to the Harvard undergraduates. Bigelow, listening to this eloquent man, realized that it would be possible - following the obvious example of Warren - to become an educated and accomplished citizen of the city of Boston as a physician.

George Edward Ellis (1814-1894), a Unitarian minister who left the ministry to devote himself to historical studies, became president of the Massachusetts Historical Society in 1885. In his 1880 *Memoir of Jacob Bigelow, M.D., LL.D.*, he wrote,

> The eminent and gifted Dr. John Warren...began to deliver lectures on anatomy to the senior class in college, and was next year made Professor of Anatomy. Dr. Bigelow used often through the remainder of his life to speak in glowing and delightful language of the power and fluency and eloquence with which Dr. Warren lectured, wholly without notes. It seems to have been through the charm and sway of this eminent anatomist that our subject was won to his profession.[1]

This was all very well and good, but Bigelow had no money and was out on his own at the age of nineteen. Without the means to continue his education, he taught in a boys' school in Worcester for a year, a very common interim profession for men at that time.

In 1808 Bigelow returned to Boston to study medicine. He attended the lectures given in Cambridge by three professors, John Warren (Anatomy), Aaron Dexter (Chemistry), and Benjamin Waterhouse

(Theory and Practice of Physic). These lecture courses lasted from four to six months, and were given for two years. There was apparently little, if any, anatomical, laboratory, or clinical exposure for the students. The Massachusetts General Hospital would not be built for another ten years. According to custom, Bigelow apprenticed himself as a pupil to Dr. John Gorham, a young and bright physician who was also a lecturer on chemistry and a physician to several of the city charities.

Essentially without funds to support himself, Bigelow found a position as assistant teacher at the Public Latin School which he held for a year and a half. It is instructive for us to know that he also intentionally used this time to improve his own skills in classical Latin and Greek, noting that the best learning comes through teaching; this saying is as valid today as in all our previous years. His classical interests persisted throughout his lifetime and he found them supportive of both his personal and his professional lives.

In 1808 Bigelow received his Master's degree with honors; his prize was writing and reciting a poem. Harvard did not award an M.D. degree until 1810, after the University of Pennsylvania began to do so the year before. Cambridge was not to be outdone by Philadelphia! In fact, Bigelow, realizing the inadequate education he received, went to Philadelphia in 1809 to continue his studies. It is most revealing of the intellectual and personal character of Bigelow to know that one of his teachers there was Benjamin Rush, the proponent of bloodletting as the effective treatment for almost every disease. Bigelow was also a pupil of Dr. Benjamin Smith Barton, a botanist who instilled in him a lifelong interest in the study of plants, both for pleasure and for potential therapeutic value. Bigelow earned his M.D. degree in 1810 and returned to Boston to open his office practice on Orange Street. Earlier, in 1803, the Boylston Fund of five hundred dollars had been established, the interest of which was to be awarded for the best essay on a medical topic. Bigelow won this prize three times in 1811 and 1812 for his papers written on medical conditions: a throat disease (Cynanche maligna), phthysis (tuberculosis), and the treatment of burns.

On his return to Boston Bigelow was quick to renew his friendships with old friends, classmates, and instructors. He was invited to join a half-dozen men who met regularly on Saturday evenings at the home of George Ticknor where they discussed the literature of the day: Scott, Crabbe, Byron, and others. Their notes were written in Latin, and they had a fine time together. There was also the Anthology Club, organized in 1805 that met weekly, fourteen men devoted to developing the literary talent that they felt was latent in Boston. These men would work together over the years to develop reading rooms, literary journals, and an excellent library, the Boston Athenaeum. These friendships and the writings Bigelow did for the Boylston prizes were, for him, steps up a ladder that he felt to be essential for his life. He knew that success in his professional life was dependent upon becoming a member of the inner circle of the city's medical and social world. This was accomplished for him when, in 1811, he was asked to become a partner of Dr. James Jackson, by far and away the leading physician in the city. Jackson had been appointed Professor of Theory and Practice at Harvard and wanted some free time to prepare his lectures. Their friendship and professional relations prospered over the next fifty years; Bigelow would succeed Jackson as President of the Massachusetts Medical Society and as President of the American Academy of Arts and Sciences.

The Academic Career

An interest in botany, begun as a child and encouraged during his time at Philadelphia with Dr. Barton, led him to inquire about offering a public lecture series on the subject in 1812. This was instigated by learning that Dr. John Gorham, the physician whose apprentice-pupil Bigelow had been, was delivering a popular lecture series on chemistry. Bigelow conferred with John Lowell, a prominent barrister, who referred him to William D. Peck who had been asked to do such a series. The two worked together and this was the beginning of what would be a second career for Bigelow. The interest of the students was impressive and led Bigelow to publish, in 1814, his first book, *Florula Bostoniensis.* There were subsequent editions that extended the survey farther, and, until 1848 with the publication of Asa Gray's work, this study was the standard reference for herborists in New England. Bigelow also illustrated his book with colored engravings that he taught himself to make. Certainly a major influence of his book was his substitution of generic names for the Latin ones, making ready access to the text practical. This book on Boston flowers became known across the United States and Europe, and a lifetime of correspondence developed with natural scientists and botanists here and abroad who shared his interests and concerns.

In 1815 Bigelow was appointed Lecturer in Materia Medica and Botany at Harvard, the beginning of his academic career. The following year he was appointed Rumford Professor at Harvard. Count

Rumford was born Benjamin Thompson in Woburn, Massachusetts in 1753. He was an active proponent of his own welfare, becoming wealthy as a young man. He was knighted by George III for his work for the British Army during the Revolutionary War. He did, however, have a dedicated interest in the needs of the poor, working in various European countries on their behalf. One of his ongoing concerns was the need to teach what would be called, the Sciences of the Useful Arts. At his death near Paris in 1814, he left his estate to Harvard to establish a lecture professorship to be called, The Rumford Professor of the Application of Science to the Useful Arts. Bigelow was chosen as the first Rumford Professor to deliver these lectures.

James Gregory Mumford, a prominent Boston surgeon and medical historian, in his lecture on Jacob Bigelow before the Johns Hopkins Hospital Historical Club on October 14, 1901, said,

> I think that this appointment, and the meaning of it all, came to be for Bigelow the most significant event of his life. Doubtless, the developing science of the last century would have found in him an enthusiastic student under any circumstances. But it is fair to suppose that Rumford...left behind in his native State a young disciple, who needed only that brilliant and successful example to lead him wisely toward the pursuit of truth.[2]

This effusive language is important for understanding the career of Bigelow. He very early took a stand in favor of education in technology as he watched the economic growth of the United States in industries. He would continue to support the education and training of engineers, scientists, artisans, architects, and many more that he readily accepted into the category of 'profession,' expanding the original restriction to the classical ones of law, clergy, and medicine.

A side note on the initiation of the Rumford lectureship is important in understanding the changes about to occur in American education. There was an academic uproar, particularly in the English universities and in Edinburgh, decrying what seemed to reviewers to be an abandonment of the standard classical education in favor of what would subsequently be called, technology. The lectures by Bigelow demonstrated clearly to the British professors that academic life had deteriorated. John Adams, the former President of the United States, wrote to Bigelow applauding his efforts and commenting on the reviewers.

> Accept my thanks for your Inaugural Oration....The Edinburgh Reviewers have said that "if the whole of American literature were annihilated, with the exception perhaps of something of Franklin, the world would lose

nothing of the useful or agreeable.
Your inaugural discourse, Mr. Bigelow, is a sufficient refutation of that
puerile flight of those great men. You may challenge the three kingdoms
to produce a character, in the last hundred years, more useful to his species
than the founder of your professorship.[3]

Bigelow would continue to work towards educational goals that
recognized that there was more to education than a reading knowledge
of Greek and Latin. He continued to give the annual Rumford lectures
until 1827, when he retired from the professorship. In 1829 he
published the first edition of *Elements of Technology,* a 500 page
discourse, based on his lectures, that cover an astounding variety of the
sciences of technology: printing, clock making, architecture, engraving,
water supply, ventilation, and many others. A second edition appeared
two years later. Another delightful side note is that Bigelow was
attacked for his lecture because he was an *insider,* one who knew the
classics. How could he betray his commitment to his own kind?

In 1817 Bigelow was promoted to professor of Materia Medica, a
position he held until 1855. But his interest in botany continued to be a
strong influence on his work. In 1818 he began publication of a three-
volume *American Medical Botany* that he illustrated himself, struggling
to develop the right techniques for color printing and engraving. He
found the professional printers inadequate, so he devised his own
methods that were successful. He produced sixty plates and sixty
thousand colored engravings for the work. Again, his simplification of
terms and clarity of writing, combined with an exquisite attention to
details of weather, temperature, wind direction, and rainfall, made
these books of great value to gardeners.

In 1820 Bigelow was one of a committee of five men who brought
out the first edition of the *Pharmacopoeia of the United States.* Again,
an important part of this work was the simplification of terms, making
the book readily accessible to its users. Commenting later on the
usefulness of the text, Bigelow wrote that

This simple and convenient nomenclature continues to be used in this
country, and seems likely in time to supersede all others, at least so long as
medicine continues to be made a mystery, and pharmacy a trade, and
therapeutics almost a pseudo-science.[4]

Bigelow later published a summary of the *Materia Medica,* the
practical section that would be of use to practitioners that was known
as "Bigelow's Sequel."

Cholera

In 1832 cholera appeared in New York City in epidemic form; the final death count was 3000. The Board of the Commissioners of Health of Boston appointed Bigelow, John Ware, and Joshua B. Flint to visit New York to ascertain the nature of the disease and report back to them about measures they might take to prevent an epidemic. The experience was frightening for Bigelow: the streets were empty of people and of conveyances, the healthy having left the city. The sick were poorly treated, nurses having also fled. Bigelow was cheered to find that the doctors were still at the hospitals caring, as best they could, for the victims. On their return to Boston by steamboat, health authorities in Providence forbid their entry into the city; they landed at Seekonk and took a stage coach home. Their report to the mayor and the Board was so terrifying in its description of their visit that the Board decided not to publish it, apparently fearful of the terror it might incite. In Boston, there were 100 deaths from cholera.

This experience, and a paper published thirty-four years later in the *Boston Medical and Surgical Journal,* offer the reader an instructive view of both commitment to the sick and human fallibility in understanding what lies right in front of us. Although Bigelow does not mention it in his personal notes, several of his colleagues had refused to go on the mission. He found this distressing due to his conviction that the physician is required to care for the sick, no matter how serious or dangerous the infection is; the only caveat is to not carry the disease to others.

The paper written by Bigelow is instructive for all students because it points out the fact that our learning is an ongoing process and we must be cautious in stating that certain conditions, arrangements, observations, and experiences are true. Not all of his ideas and opinions reflect his own avowed reliance on scientific reasoning, an observation essential to our own education and training. There is a common tendency - regardless of the year in history - to assume that we do, finally, in our time and place, know what we are doing. Our scientific foundation is reliable, our observations are accurate and verifiable, and our reasoning is sound. We forget that we must maintain a most modest posture about the sufficiency's of the art of medicine and the limits of our scientific expertise.

Bigelow would certainly have agreed with this position in his day, and he supported it in the 1866 article referred to above, "Whether Cholera is Contagious." In this paper he describes the geographic spread of cholera, both in 1831-32 and 1847, pointing out that the mode of travel of the disease is not known. He noted that we know as much about how the disease spreads as we knew about lightning before we knew about electricity. He continued, in his paper:

> Its conveyance and propagation have been ascribed to air, to water, to material foci, to electricity, to ozone or to the want of it. Of late, in consequence of the vast development by the microscope of the existence everywhere of minute living organisms, it has become more common to ascribe the arrival of this and other like epidemics to certain unseen "germs" which are called seeds or ova, cryptogamic or animalcular, according as the fancy of the theorist inclines him to adopt a vegetable or an animal nomenclature.[5]

It is amazing to read this, knowing it was written some seventeen years after John Snow was awarded the prize from the Institute of Paris for showing that cholera is carried in water, and twelve years after the vestrymen of St. James removed the handle of the Broad Street pump, halting the epidemic in that section of London.

Bigelow accepted contagion as a cause of some diseases such as smallpox, but denied it here. He clearly placed the causes of cholera in the socioeconomic status of its victims. Poor sanitation, dirt, poverty and overcrowding were essential for the appearance and the spread of this disease. His advice to his readers was reassuring.

> People who would avoid or prevent cholera should cultivate equanimity, regularity of life and habits, cleanliness, salubrious exercise, temperance, and avoidance of all excesses. When they have done their duty in providing for the care of the sick, allaying public panics, and abating public nuisances, they may safely dismiss their apprehensions.[6]

As I noted above, our lessons from this outstanding physician and public figure should include humility before our tasks and our skills, and gratitude for our opportunities to learn. The discovery of the anthrax bacillus by Robert Koch was only a decade away, and his announcement of the bacterial cause of tuberculosis would appear in 1882. At the time Bigelow was writing this paper on cholera, Louis Pasteur was working on the causes of fermentation in wine and the souring of milk. In 1881 he would vaccinate sheep against anthrax, and, in 1885, a boy against rabies.

Rational Medicine

In 1833 Bigelow and his wife made their first trip to Italy. They were accompanied by a group of Bostonians, one of whom was Oliver Wendell Holmes. A recent graduate of Harvard Medical School, Holmes was on his way to study at the Paris Clinical School. Bigelow was introduced by James Jackson, Jr., son of the renowned Boston physician and partner of Bigelow, to a number of the French physicians who were faculty members of the School. Their new way of looking at the practice of medicine through empiricism, statistical analysis, and pathological study was having a impressive and visible impact on young American doctors who went to Paris to study. For Bigelow, the teachings of Pierre Louis were tranformingly important: particularly his analysis of venesection for the treatment of pneumonia. Louis had shown that bloodletting had very limited - if any - therapeutic effect on that disease. As Bigelow thought through his own experiences in practice, his lectures to students on the need to observe carefully, and questions on the efficacy of drugs raised by his botanical and pharmacological studies, he came more and more to doubt a lot of the therapies prescribed by doctors.

In keeping with our propensity to construct a rationale for what we see in the world, the history, both of medicine and of the sciences, is replete with explanations for diseases and their treatments, usually spun out of thin air. Early in Bigelow's career he was convinced on the need to observe as carefully as one could before drawing any conclusions. As J.G. Mumford wrote, in his lecture at Hopkins,

> In those early days, when ingenious men were advancing theories founded on speculation and insufficient observation; when text-books were loaded with *ex cathedra* dicta, dogmatic teachers were looked up to by the public and medical students as almost divine healers.[7]

In the early years of the nineteenth century physicians relied on the authority of what were knows as 'Systems,' intellectual constructs that defined diagnosis and treatment. These systems were also labeled as being 'rational,' as being reasonable for the understanding of both patient and doctor. It is important, in understanding the teachings of Bigelow, to know this category of medical reasoning because Bigelow would use the word, rational, in his writings to mean, not a system of medicine, but the use of the human faculty of reason to understand what one does in life and in work. We will return to this discussion below.

In 1835 Bigelow delivered "A Discourse on Self-Limited Diseases" before the annual meeting of the Massachusetts Medical Society. This lecture was the result of his thinking through the work of the Paris School, his own experiences in practice and in teaching, and his observations of the natural history of disease. This landmark essay was called by Ellis, "the most important and striking paper," and a "remarkable, and at the time of its delivery, startling production."[8] This was a watershed moment in American medicine, one that changed both the understanding of diseases and their treatments. Coming, as it did, at a time of dissatisfaction of the public with medical care, careful attention was paid to it. Oliver Wendell Holmes noted the impact of Bigelow's lecture in his retrospective 1879 report to the Council of the American Academy of Arts and Sciences following the death of Bigelow. Holmes wrote,

> This remarkable essay has probably had more influence on medical practice in America than any similar brief treatise, we might say than any other work, ever published in this country....Dr. Bigelow's discourse summed up the question between nature and medical art so clearly, that from that day forward the empirical habit of interference, for the sake of interfering, with the course of a self-evolving and self-terminating disease may be said to have declined.[9]

What had Bigelow done? In a remarkably reasoned and understandable way he divided diseases into three categories within which he discussed principles of treatment: 1), self-limited, 2), curable, and 3), incurable diseases. A self-limited disease is

> one which, after it has obtained foothold in the system, cannot, in the present state of our knowledge, be eradicated, or abridged, by art, - but to which there is due a certain succession of processes, to be completed in a certain time; which time and processes may vary with the constitution and condition of the patient, and may tend to death or to recovery, but are not known to be shortened, or greatly changed, by medical treatment.[10]

Bigelow was initiating the movement in American medicine, later to be labeled "therapeutic nihilism," that called into radical question the value of the nostrums and heroic measures common to medical practice. The vast number of drugs, the continued use of venesection, emetics, and purgatives, plus the obvious turn of the people toward alternative, or irregular, healers made physicians increasingly aware of the need for accurate diagnosis and attention to the needs of the patient. *Caring* for patients became a recommended practice.

Bigelow, in his description of self-limited diseases, was not recommending ignoring the patient. He continued, in his essay,

These expressions are not intended to apply to the palliation of diseases, for he who turns a pillow, or administers a seasonable draught of water to a patient, palliates his suffering; but they apply to the more important consideration of removing diseases themselves through medical means.[11]

His argument continued as he pointed out the failures of doctors to prove the existence of effective remedies for most diseases. This observation was, of course, an underlying conviction of all those patients who sought herbalists, homeopaths, Mesmerism, and the other alternative healers. Bigelow sealed his argument by noting that doctors die of the diseases they attempt to cure! He was concerned with the search for truth as the foundation of knowledge. He wrote,

For truth then, we must earnestly seek, even when its developments do not flatter our professional pride, nor attest the infallibility of our art....Independently of the common defects of medical evidence, our self-interest, our self-esteem, and sometimes even our feelings of humanity may be arrayed against the truth.[12]

Physicians must be cautious in treatment lest they interfere with healing accomplished by Nature; the art of medicine may damage more than assist. Bigelow asserted that

We may do much good by a palliative, and preventive course, by alleviating pain, procuring sleep, guarding the diet, regulating the alimentary tract, - in fine, by obviating such suffering as admits of mitigation, and preventing, or removing the causes of others, which are incidental, but not necessary, to the state of disease. In doing this, we must distinguish between the disease itself, and the accidents of the disease, for the latter often admit of relief, when the former do not.[13]

I have used extended quotations from this 1835 address because it was a seminal moment, calling into question many of the foundations of practice taught in medical schools. It is important to recall that these were the years of the explosion in proprietary schools that offered no clinical training, relying entirely on brief series of lectures and a few textbooks. The central tenet of Bigelow's thesis is the necessity for accurate diagnosis made through observation: impeccable detailing of the medical history and examination of the patient. It is important for us to recognize our feet of clay: in a lecture to the entering class at the medical school twenty years later, Bigelow agreed with current thought that, in some cases of inflammatory disease, bloodletting was of value, at least early in the course of the illness.

On Education

As one reads through the papers and addresses that Bigleow prepared during the long course of his professional life, it becomes clear that, for acute observers of the scene, the central problem to be confronted in American medicine was proper education and training of medical students. There was an obvious need to reconsider how students were taught, and what they were taught. The American Medical Association, founded in 1847, was struggling with these problems and, in 1850, Bigelow submitted a short paper to the membership, "Practical Views on Medical Education." In this paper he discussed the varied fundamentals of a medical education - chemistry, anatomy, materia medica, surgery, and obstetrics, and others. He deplored the excessive focus on therapeutics, noting that students often came away with the conviction that there was a drug for every disease and every symptom. His concerns were with the teachers.

> Much injury is done to the cause of true learning by medical assumption, amplification, and exaggeration, by premature adoption of novelties, and by tenacity of theories, personal or espoused. Students, in all former years, have expended much time in learning what it afterwards cost them both time and trouble to unlearn,....[14]

Bigelow pressed for a three-year course of study that was based upon the elementary principles of the sciences, that urged thoughtful inquiry by students into their reasoning in the care of patients, and demanded faithfulness to the protracted and methodical study required of them for the rest of their careers. Bigelow closed his article with this advice.

> The things to be avoided by medical teachers are technicalities, which are unintelligible to beginners; gratuitous assumptions, and citations of doubtful authorities; prolix dissertations on speculative topics; excessive minuteness in regard to subjects which are intricate and but little used, and therefore destined to be speedily forgotten. To these may be added controversies, superfluous personal eulogiums and criminations, and all self-exaggeration, personal or local.[15]

There is an uncanny ring to these words when we look at medical education in our contemporary era. There remains the need for attending to the very cautions Bigelow outlined 150 years ago. He was seeking for a framework for teaching young men, not only the fundamentals of the limited sciences of the time, but also the interior structure that the physician needs in order to practice properly. In 1852 Bigelow gave the Introductory Address to the medical students at the Massachusetts Medical College (Harvard). They were so impressed that they asked his permission to publish it. In this paper Bigelow spoke of his earlier work on self-limited diseases, and then went on to discuss the medical profession as an inexact science when compared to mathematics and astronomy. While some men pursue the exact sciences, most choose to work in the areas of uncertainty and conjecture. He called the attention of the students to the fact that,

> Preeminent among the inexact and speculative sciences stands *practical medicine,* a science older than civilization, cultivated and honored in all ages, powerful for good or for evil, progressive in its character, but still unsettled in its principles; remunerative in fame and fortune to its successful cultivators, and rich in the fruits of a good conscience to its honest votaries. Encumbered as it is with difficulty, fallacy and doubt, medicine yet constitutes one of the most attractive of the learned professions.[16]

In keeping with his growing concern for the inadequacies of medical education and practice and the current focus on therapeutics by herbalists and regular physicians alike, Bigelow went on to stress for the students his definition of the good doctor, in *italics,* at that.

> If the question be asked, what makes a great physician, and one who is appealed to by his peers, and by the discerning portion of the public, for counsel in difficult cases, I would answer, that *he is a great physician who, above other men, understands diagnosis.*[17]

Bigelow pressed the students to beware of theories that lacked scientific proof, and of making claims about medical accomplishments that could not be sustained by the evidence. He was moving steadily toward a revision of the definition of the good doctor at a time when public doubts were fully reflected in the steady rise of alternative methods of treatment across the nation.

The confusions about the terms used to define the varied methods of medical theory and practice - system, rational, empiric, sectarianism, and specifics - were clarified by Bigelow in an address he gave before the Massachusetts Medical Society in 1858. He called his address, *Expositions of Rational Medicine,* and in it he defined five distinct methods by which medicine was practiced in America. Briefly, his presentation can be presented as:

1. The Artificial Method was based upon the treatment of symptoms, essentially ignoring the diagnosis. This method reached its epitome in 'heroics' where inflammation and fever were treated by purging and bleeding; wasting and fatigue by stimulants and alcohol.

2. The Expectant Method relied on nature to heal, using the examples of animals and native tribes that recover without treatment. Although it was admitted that doctors may have done more damage than disease over all these centuries, Bigelow believed that thoughtful physicians could help.

3. Homeopathy was considered a variation on the expectant method, one that Bigelow thought would end up in the category of 'historical delusions.' He did note its corrective to heroic therapies.

4. The Exclusive Method was one that relied on a single treatment scheme: hydrotherapy, mineral spirits, exercise, electricity, magnets, and other specious techniques were included.

5. The Rational Method is, of course, the one espoused by Bigelow originally in his address on self-limited diseases. Accurate diagnosis, appropriate treatment, and care of the patient are the hallmarks of this reasoned approach to medicine. In his description of this method, obviously his choice, Bigelow wrote that

> Our present defect is not that we know too little, but that we profess too much....It is the part of rational medicine to study intelligently the nature, degree and tendency, of each existing case, and afterwards to act, or to forbear acting, as the exigencies of each case may require. To do all this wisely and efficiently, the practitioner must possess, first, sufficient knowledge to diagnosticate the disease; and, secondly, sufficient sense as well as knowledge to make up a correct judgment on the course to be pursued.[18]

The use of reason - the Rational Method - as the proper way to practice medicine opened, for Bigelow and his enthusiastic students, the way to truly care for patients. He was certainly aware of the inadequacies of the sciences that medicine hoped to rely upon: chemistry, physics, microscopy, experimental physiology. They were in their infancy in his time. But he was also alert to the need to care for persons who were ill. In his paper on Rational Medicine, quoted above, he uses the very apt phrase, "safe conduct of the sick" to define the role of the physician.[19]

Bigelow had earlier on made a bad name for himself with the classicists, those professors in the United States, but particularly in England, whose definition of the educated included only those who had studied the ancients and mastered Greek and Latin. Bigelow, as stated so clearly in his Rumford lectures, was a strong advocate of advanced education for the new professions such as engineering, architecture, mechanics, and metallurgy. He stressed also the importance of assuring youth that learning a trade and becoming a valued citizen with reading and writing skills were goals worthy of them; useful labor was honorable. In the period of rapid industrial and agricultural growth in America that followed upon the Civil War, education would not be defined only by a working knowledge of the classics; there was a modern wisdom to be mastered.

In 1861 the State of Massachusetts incorporated a new institution, the Massachusetts Institute of Technology in Cambridge. The word, technology, was almost an invention of Bigelow himself, not appearing in dictionaries before his time. As one of the memorable events of his life, he was invited to deliver an address at the opening of the Institute in its new building on November 16, 1865. His *Address on the Limits of Education* is an engaging paper. Speaking to the meaning of education, he noted that "A common college education now culminates in the student becoming what is called a master of arts. But this in a majority of instances means simply a master of nothing."[20]

The graduate, to move on and earn a living would, of necessity, have to receive some training.

M.I.T. would be the school that would teach the special branches of useful knowledge, fitting in with the amazing new needs of a growing country. Bigelow did not deny the pleasures of a classical education; he [21]just found it to be a luxury, producing men capable of becoming orators and writers. What the world demands now is

a better citizen, a more sagacious statesman, a more far-sighted economist, a more able financier, a more skilful engineer, manufacturer, merchant, or military commander....Antiquity has produced many great men. Modern times have produced equally great men, and more of them.[22]

Bigelow made an effort, in this talk, to instill a love of learning that would inform a generation of men who would be witnesses to the forthcoming era of industrialization. Learning was important, regardless of the field.

Knowledge is never so successfully cultivated as when it becomes a pleasure, and no pleasure is more permanent than the successful pursuit of knowledge, combined, as it should be, with moral progress.[23]

Bigelow received considerable correspondence castigating him for what were interpreted as negative comments on the value of a classical education. He took these without rancor, confident that his own superb education in the classics and his prestige as a renowned physician and advocate for improved education would carry him through.

Commentary

Jacob Bigelow was a key figure in American medicine in his time. He knew the radical changes in medicine that were effected by the teachings of the Paris School, more and more apparent as hundreds - later thousands - of doctors went to Paris and later to Germany to learn the new sciences of medicine. Bigelow was also aware that the changes in medicine reflected on his own past ignorance, and he was humble before this knowledge. He realized that changes would be a constant. He helped the profession reassess its roles in caring for patients, encouraging a more modest posture toward the power of the doctor to cure. In his 1852 lecture to the medical students, quoted above, he said,

> Most men form an exaggerated estimate of the powers of medicine, founded on the common acceptation of the name, that medicine is the art of curing disease. That this is a false definition is evident from the fact that many diseases are incurable, and that one such disease must at last happen to every living man. A far more just definition would be, that medicine is the art of understanding diseases, and of curing or relieving them when possible. Under this acceptation our science would, at least, be exonerated from reproach, and would stand on a basis capable of supporting a reasonable and durable system for the amelioration of human maladies.[24]

Bigelow offered a reasoned and gentle approach to the reform of American medicine, so needed at the time.

Friends and colleagues were important to Bigelow and he kept in touch with college friends who shared his interests in classical poetry, botany, and the general welfare of Boston. He was also an accomplished artist; his botanical illustrations drew the applause of Thomas Jefferson and Asa Gray, the renowned Harvard Darwinian botanist. An amazing and unexpected finding was revealed when a number of Bigelow's friends received a book with the title, *Eolopoesis: American Rejected Addresses.* It was published in 1855 and was addressed to the Directors of the New York Crystal Palace. It was a collection of sixteen humorous poems about famous literary and historical figures of the past, each of whom had a secret. Each poem concluded with the initials of an outstanding contemporary American writer: Emerson, Lowell, Holmes, Longfellow, and others. It was, of course, a joke, and was received appropriately by the supposed authors. Bigelow was well aware of the changes occurring in his world, the new industrial age following on the end of the Civil War. His life presents an opportunity for physicians to learn about their careers as persons constantly learning. For not all his ideas and opinions reflect his own avowed commitments to truth and to scientific reasoning. He wrote to the *Boston Daily Advertiser* in 1862,

> We are discovering at last that the South are a dangerous people. Warlike, audacious, needy, unscrupulous, individually disinclined and disqualified for industrial pursuits, but both inclined and qualified for war, rapine, and conquest, their separate existence in incompatible with the peace of the world.[25]

This observation is essential for contemporary training and education. There is a common tendency to assume that we do, finally, in our time and place, know what we are doing; our scientific foundation is reliable, our observations are accurate and verifiable, and our reasoning is sound. We so easily forget that we must maintain a modest posture about the sufficiencies of the art of medicine and the limits of our expertise.

Bigelow would have agreed in his day. His stand on the contagiousness of cholera is a notable example that would have humbled him. Another arresting article by Bigelow is one written for the *American Journal of Medical Sciences* in 1852. Questions had been raised about the safety of water brought to Boston in lead pipes. As a member of the committee asked to investigate, Bigelow felt there was no danger, even though lead was obtained from the water after evaporation. Bigelow pointed to the ubiquity of lead in paint, furniture, buckets, chest linings, and other devices; he decided that cases of encephalopathy, lead colic, and arthralgia were coincidental, not causally related to the water supply. Bigelow compared the risk of traveling by ship and railroad, being exposed to fire, drink and medicine, and wrote that, "it is not probable that the leaden aqueduct will be abandoned on account of the inconsiderable risk which it may involve of occasioning disease."[26]

George Ellis interviewed Bigelow near the end of his life. He had been blind for five years and was bedridden with some type of paralysis. In his Memoir of Bigelow, Ellis wrote,

> The answers were often communicative, and generally toned in humor and drollery. As, for instance, to the question how, in the lack of all our

modern means in medical schools, hospitals, &c., he obtained his first professional training and knowledge, he replied, "Oh, from my patients."[27]

This is still a central part of the learning experience for the medical student and the practitioner. The career of Bigelow presents an opportunity to learn about the paths our own careers will follow, be they in the academy, in the laboratory, or in the practice of medicine. He ended his career respected and appreciated for his many skills in the practice of medicine, his writings, and his teachings. His wide-ranging interests in art, technology, the classics, and his critical approach to education make him a teacher for all students who seek knowledge and the eternally valid posture of questioning what is taken for truth. As Henry David Thoreau wrote, "Any truth is better than make-believe."[28]

----

[1]Ellis, George E., Memoir of Jacob Bigelow, M.D., LL.D., Cambridge, John Wilson and Son, University Press, 1880, 19.
[2]Mumford, J.G., JACOB BIGELOW-A SKETCH, Johns Hopkins Hospital Bulletin. vol. XIII, No. 130, January, 1902, 3.
[3]Ellis, op. cit., 46-47.
[4]Ellis, Ibid., 54.
[5]Bigelow, Jacob, "Whether Cholera is Contagious," Modern Inquiries: Classical, Professional, and Miscellaneous, Boston, Little, Brown, and Company, 1873, 290.
[6]Bigelow, Ibid., 293-294.
[7]Mumford, op. cit., 13.
[8]Ellis, op. cit., 77.
[9]Holmes, Oliver Wendell, "Report of the Council," American Academy of Arts and Sciences, May 27, 1879.
[10]Bigelow, Jacob, Discourse on Self-Limited Diseases, Boston, Nathan Hale...Water Street, 1835, 8-9.
[11]Ibid., 9.
[12]Ibid., 26-27.
[13]Ibid., 33-34.
[14]Bigelow, Jacob, "Practical Views on Medical Education," Modern Inquiries: Classical, Professional and Miscellaneous, Boston, Little, Brown, and Company, 1870, 266-267.
[15]Ibid., 270.
[16]Bigelow, Jacob, A Lecture on the Treatment of Disease, Boston, Ticknor, Reed, and Fields, 1853, 7.
[17]Ibid., 11.
[18]Bigelow, Jacob, Brief Expositions of Rational Medicine, Boston, Phillips, Sampson and Company, 1858, 48, 50-51.
[19]Ibid., 33.

[20]Bigelow, Jacob, An Address on the Limits of Education, Boston, E. P. Dutton & Company, 1865, 15.

[21]

[22]Ibid., 17-18.

[23]Ibid., 26.

[24]Bigelow, Jacob, op. cit., On the Treatment..., 9.

[25]Bigelow, Jacob, "The Dark Side, The Bright Side, the Practible Side," in *Modern Inquiries:...,* op cit., 371.

[26]Bigelow, Jacob, "Report on the Action of Cochituate Water on Lead Pipes; and the Influence of the Same on Health," American Journal of Medical Sciences, 1852, in Nature and Disease, Boston, Ticknor and Fields, MDCCCLIV, 322.

[27]Ellis, op. cit., 7.

[28]Thoreau, Henry David, Walden, edited by J. Lyndon Shanley, Princeton, Princeton University Press, 1971, 327.

Chapter 4

John Young Bassett, 1805-1851

The biographical narrative about this Alabama physician is remarkable in that it became available to us through a series of coincidences. Bassett's life, cut short at the age of 46 years by tuberculosis, was like many other doctors who practiced in the United States at the time. He received the typical limited education that was available in the first third of the nineteenth century, set up his practice in Huntsville, Alabama, married and had children, and practiced pretty much the same style of medicine as the other doctors in Madison County. He did go to Paris to study in 1836, an experience I will detail shortly. The life-drama of Doctor Bassett has four actors in it who tell our story. But we would know nothing of him had it not been for the remarkable inquisitiveness of the premier physician in the English speaking world at the close of the nineteenth century - William Osler.

William Osler

In what would become one of his most popular essays, *An Alabama Student,* published in 1896, Osler told of his discovery of Bassett. The preceding year he presented the paper as a talk before the Johns Hopkins Hospital Historical Club, introducing his subject thus:

> Tonight I wish to tell you the story of a man of whom you have never heard, whose name is not written on the scroll of fame, but of one who heard the call and forsook all and followed his ideal.[1]

Osler was doing some research on malarial fevers in the South. In his reading, he came across two volumes of the *Southern Medical Reports* for the years 1849-50 and 1850-51, the only two issues of that journal ever published. Osler, impressed in reading two essays by a Dr. John Y. Bassett of Huntsville, Alabama, found in him one "in whom I seemed to recognize a 'likeness to the wise below', a 'kindred with the great of old'."[2] The crucial part of this encounter was the display of a personal and professional characteristic that made Osler a renowned doctor, teacher, and scholar of medical history: his curiosity, so readily aroused, that made pursuit of knowledge imperative. Osler wrote to an acquaintance in Huntsville to find out what had become of Dr. Bassett. His inquiry was referred to Dr. Bassett's daughter who forwarded a collection of letters that Bassett had written at the time of his trip to Paris. These letters offered Osler insights into a man about whom he wrote,

> There are a few men in every community who, from temperment or conviction, cannot bow to the Baals of the society about them, and who stand aloof, in thought at least, from the common herd. Such men tread a steep and thorny road, and of such in all ages has the race delighted to make martyrs. The letters indicate in Dr. Bassett a restless, nonconforming spirit, which turned aside from the hollowness and deceit of much of the life about him.[3]

Bassett's letters are currently in the Alabama Department of Archives and History in Montgomerey. I will return to some of the interpretations and comments of Osler later.

Erasmus Darwin Fenner

The second man who forms the backdrop for this study was the editor of the *Southern Medical Reports,* Erasmus Darwin Fenner. A native of North Carolina, he graduated from Transylvania and settled in New Orleans in 1841. A firm believer in the inherent differences between medical conditions and practice in the North and in the South, he was instrumental in the publication of several medical journals. He began publication of the *New Orleans Medical Journal* in 1841. In 1856 he helped form the New Orleans School of Medicine, and became Dean of the Faculty and held the chair of Principles and Practice. Of note about this school is the fact that the first medical student clerkship program was begun here. Also, despite anxieties about losing students, the course of study was lengthened. Fenner believed, as did Bassett, in what was called, "the unity of the fevers," i.e., the treatment of symptoms - regardless of the disease - was the same: bleeding, purging, cold baths, and other nostrums. Fenner placed considerable importance on the roles of climate and meteorology in causing illness, and requested physicians to document the conditions in their locales and forward their findings to him for publication. Thus did the writings of Bassett become known to Osler and then to us.

Claudius H. Mastin

Osler read his paper, "An Alabama Student," before the January 1895 meeting of the Johns Hopkins Hospital Historical Club, and it was published a year later in the January 1896 issue of the *Johns Hopkins Hospital Bulletin,* number 58. The following April Claudius H. Mastin, M.D., a physician in Mobile, Alabama, heard about Osler's paper from a friend and wrote to Osler to offer him some additional information about Bassett to which Osler was not privy. Mastin wrote,

> Having decided to make Medicine my profession, I looked around for a preceptor who would mark out the proper course for me to take, and after due investigation, I concluded that Dr. John Y. Bassett was, by all odds, the best fitted man in that town to give me the instruction I required. Thus it was that I entered his office as a pupil in 1846 and remained with him for eighteen months, when he advised me to go to the University of Pennsylvania and gave me a letter of introduction to his personal friend Prof. Geo. B. Wood.[4]

This letter to Osler provided some details that present a fuller picture of the personal and the professional life of Bassett.

John Young Bassett

John Young Bassett was born in Baltimore, Maryland. He was one of seven children, of whom five survived infancy. Emmett B. Carmichael, in a 1964 paper on Bassett, wrote,

> The third son, John Young, was of a different temperment from his two older brothers. He was quiet, more studious, graver, more sober, and much gentler with his mother than the older brothers. John stayed at home and from early childhood he expressed a desire to become a musician.[5]

His oldest brother, a surgeon in the U.S. Navy, was killed in a duel in Rio de Janiero; his younger brother, Frank, would die of tetanus in Huntsville after a shooting accident. His sister, whom I will return to, was an unhappy woman. Their father died in his forties, and the boys went to work to support the family. John became an apprentice to a druggist in Baltimore, working by day and studying by night. He opened his own store with a physician, which he subsequently sold to study medicine at the Washington Medical College in Baltimore; this school was founded in 1827 and Bassett received his diploma in 1828. This school would, after merging with the College of Physicians and

Surgeons of Baltimore in 1877, join the University of Maryland in 1878.

Before proceeding further with his professional life, I want to point to some revealing insights into his past found in a letter that he wrote to his wife while he was in Paris in 1836. Apparently she had written to him, concerned that she had cried in front of one of their children. He replied,

> do not weep in his presence, do not distress the poor little fellow <u>before his time</u> - for he will weep enough, and bitter enough tears, for real cause, soon enough. I remember how I was, even at his age distressed when I would think my Mother unhappy, and when I would see her weep, which was often! (for who that has raised seven children has not wept often?) I have cry'd all night long, but my infancy, <u>Isaphoena</u>, was passed in sorrow, and my boyhood without pleasure; - without sinning. I have been suffering all my life, at least until I linked my fate with yours;...[6]

This troubled heart will reappear in his professional work and his later personal life.

Bassett and his brother, Frank, an apothecary, moved to Huntsville, Alabama where they opened a drug store and John began to practice medicine. In 1831 he married Isaphoena Thompson, a daughter of a local physician; they had five children who reached maturity. Huntsville sounds like an exemplary town in which to set up a practice. It was a wealthy community; owners of plantations in Mississippi, Louisiana and southern Alabama lived there because of the climate and the educational opportunities. Sons of the town went north to Ivy League schools. Local medical care was provided by a three-man group. In his letter to Osler, Mastin wrote,

> Such was the community in which our friend had cast his fortunes: a stranger without the prestige of a name, or the influence of money, necessarily had a rough road before him; and since an influential firm, composed of Drs. Fearn, Erskine & Russel, catered to the fashion and elegance of the community, and gathered in its shekels, our friend drew his scanty support from the denizens of the hills, hollows, and caves of the surrounding country.[7]

The probable anxieties over a small practice in the rural South and a growing family, added to his expressed sadnesses of childhood and adolescence, probably contributed to his reputation in Huntsville as a difficult person. He had free time in those early years, and spent it pursuing his interests in nature and the environment. These studies would lead to his papers for Fenner's *Southern Medical Reports.* Bassett became, according to Mastin,

> an absolutely *free thinker* upon all subjects pertaining to science, politics, and religion....Our friend was considered materialistic in his views, an infidel in his belief, and as a consequence was endured rather than sustained.[8]

For reasons one can only surmise - small practice, feelings of inadequacy based upon poor medical education, or distress about lack of acceptance in the community - Bassett decided to go to Paris to study. He left Huntsville in the Fall of 1835, going by horseback via Nashville to Illinois. He stopped at Louisville, Cincinnati, and Philadelphia, finally reaching New York where, after ten days, he sailed for Liverpool. Bassett spent six weeks traveling through the cities of England, Scotland, and Ireland. In Manchester he visited a cotton factory.

> [I]t is about ten stories high & the machinery is like clock-work, one little girl will attend four looms,...I went through the Infirmary, a fine building & neatly kept; there are a great number of surgical cases in this institution in the course of a year - about 4000 were admitted last year; accidents are constantly occurring in the factories.[9]

In his visit to Edinburgh - a "City of Palaces" that he enjoyed - he watched women, called 'bearers,' employed carrying coal from the pits on their backs. A slave-owner himself, he wrote to his wife, "And this is the country that is paying Mr. Thompson to preach down American Slavery."[10] Bassett observed two operations at the Edinburgh Infirmary by Mr. William Ferguson in the presence of Mr. Syme and Sir George Bellingall: one an amputation, 'finely' done, and a plastic procedure on a deformed face. Ferguson became widely known as the founder of conservative surgery. Bassett then went on to Glasgow where he was unimpressed with the Hunterian Museum.

Paris

Bassett arrived in Paris in March 1836 and was soon introduced to the physiological studies for which the City of Lights was so renowned. In his March 11th letter to his wife he wrote,

> This morning I heard a lecture, or rather I saw Mons. Magendie (the great) experiment on living dogs, the first was a puppy about a week old, which

he literally dissected - he then bound its limbs and bound its wounds, & it walked about the table, while its mother underwent the same operation. I intend visiting very constantly the Lying-In Hospital & will become the private pupil of one of the best teachers of midwifery.[11]

Bassett was most anxious to study surgery under Velpeau and in his March 16 letter to his wife he wrote,

> Time is not wasted following Velpeau through the grand wards of La Charité, nor in hearing his lectures....From La Charité I went to the dissecting rooms, where I felt at home & have entered myself. I went to work and remained two hours....At seven I went to hear Mons. Le Doct. Helmagrand (*sic* Halma-Grand?), on midwifery; he lectured an hour, & then gives a private course on practise at his room. I also follow him, & it is my intention to put special attention to midwifery & his course is said to be good.[12]

Bassett studied with Velpeau and did well enough to be appointed an *externe* on his service - a decided honor. On July 10th Bassett wrote to his wife, "[W]hen this offer was made me I did what I have been doing all my life - made another sacrifice for my profession,...I have not been more gratified since I have been in Europe."[13]

The hospitals were readily available to foreign as well as French students and the only fees were for lectures, and they were minimal. Anatomy dissection was begun at once; subjects were very inexpensive. Bassett was given a child on his first day for forty sous. He was quite impressed with the availability of cadavers for dissection.

> There is a dissecting school at Clamart for the summer on a most extensive scale. There is room and material for 200 or upwards,...this place was provided for the inscribed students of the school, and they get their subjects for a mere trifle. There is not the least prejudice against dissections; even the subjects do not seem to mind it, though they are aware of their fate, for more that two-thirds of the dead are carried to the École Pratique or Clamart. I have private instruction in the use of the stethescope for heart complaints at La Pitié. The other day an old woman bade me adieu as we passed her bed without calling, and I stopped to ask if she was going out. Then she said she was going to Clamart, and that we might meet again.[14]

Bassett was impressed with the youthful ardor and excitement with which even the elderly mentors practiced, taught, and pursued their own studies. This was an entirely new experience for him: an environment where enthusiasm was powerful and pervasive. One of Bassett's idols in Paris was François-J.-V. Broussais, a physician who made his initial claim to fame by declaring the rational 'systems' of medicine popular in the 1820s and 1830s to be in error. John Harley Warner, commenting on the impact of this teacher, wrote,

> he was brought forward as a paragon of the French medical revolution and exemplary system-basher. But as his reputation changed both in France and in the United States, Broussaisism came to be widely regarded as the preeminent model of a rationalistic system and its attendant evils.

Warner continued with a brief summary of the medical theory of disease proposed by this physician-teacher.

> [H]e insisted on a shift in medical attention from symptoms and essentialism to lesions and localism. He denied the existence of specific diseases and held that overstimulated bodily functioning led to anatomical lesions (almost always expressed as inflammation of the gastrointestinal tract). This was the process that most diseased conditions shared, he asserted, one to be treated chiefly by local depletion using leeches.[15]

This excursus on Broussais is of interest because he was a hero for Bassett. At the very time that attendance at Broussais's lectures was shrinking rapidly, and the influence of his major antagonist, Pierre Louis, was in ascendance with Bassett's American colleagues in Paris, Bassett wrote to his sister,

> Broussais is a genius, and when he entered life he saw that something was to be done, or rather that he must do something, and he seized the Science of Medicine like a good old Doctor would a bottle of lotion, and shook it manfully....[W]hen the giant dies, I doubt if he will find a successor:...[16]

When Bassett resumed his practice in Huntsville the influence of Broussais, not of Louis or Gabriel Andral or François Chomel, would be primary in his practice.

Bassett complained to his wife that sight-seeing was rare. He did go to the Louvre, and he did see some tapestries, but this was done on the occasional Sunday when there was some time. In his April 29, 1836 letter he wrote, perhaps to justify his being in Paris in the first place,

> Some of these times I will take a few days & go round *a sight seeing* of which I have done but little since I have been here, but it must be when I have more leisure than I have at present. I am engaged every hour of the day from 7 in the morning to 9 at night. I have found much advantage in employing private instructors & paying them - it is true the courses are all public but they are crowded.[17]

Bassett continued in his letter commenting on five of his instructors in anatomy, midwifery, and surgery whom he followed diligently. His schedule was demanding. On March 26 he wrote to his wife,

> I get up in the morning at 6 o'clock & am at La Charité at seven; follow Velpeau until 8 see him operate & lecture until 1/2 after 9 - ...At 11 I am at the School of Practical Anatomie where I dissect until 2. Then I attend a class of Practice Surgery by Robier, until 3 - then hear Broussais & Andral until 5;...At seven I attend Helmagrand's class of practical Midwifery, until eleven, when I retire.[18]

Bassett, as did other American physicians who sought training in Paris, had serious questions about the moral environment of the city. There was a component to American life that was disturbed by the behavior of Parisians. Bassett found the evils in Paris to be "terrible." Writing to his wife he reflected on his past impressions of his Huntsville fellow-citizens and compared them with his current experiences. He saw himself as an "infidel" with church people at home. He wrote,

> [A]t home I looked into the evil more closely than the good effects - there I saw ignorance, bigotry & deceit ever foremost. They were the most prominent, therefore the most likely to be seen; here I still look at the evil side, & find it terrible. God save me from a country without religion; & from a government with it - ...& return me safe to a country with religion & a government without it....I am convinced that the evils of infidelity are more than any religion whatever.[19]

Another observation by Americans studying in Paris hospitals that was startling and distressing was the inhumane - occasionally even crude - behavior of physicians with their patients, especially women. French doctors did not hesitate to disrobe female patients in order to display physical signs of disease to students; they spoke openly in the presence of their patients about their poor prognosis, their expected demise and described in detail the findings anticipated at autopsy. Both the reputed New England Puritanical sense of modesty and privacy and the Southern reputation for respecting and honoring the 'weaker sex' found this Parisian professional behavior abhorrent.

When Bassett decided to go to Europe in 1835, his friends questioned this decision. He had a growing medical practice, a wife and young children, and responsibilities to his community. Bassett seemed, however, to be a very private man quite centered on his own self and its development and expression, placing the opinions of others second to his needs. From his correspondence with his wife it is apparent that they were experiencing some difficulties due to their separation. I noted this previously in discussing his letter about his childhood. In a September letter to his wife Bassett spoke to their relationship and to the impact that his time in Paris was having on both of them. He wrote, obviously in response to some comments by her, about their marriage:

> I have left you, it is true, for apparently a long time, but it is as much for your benefit as for mine. I must sustain you and to do this I must sustain myself....I used to think I was industrious & persevering, but when I look at some of the medical men by whom I am surrounded, it makes me blush for shame. Old men daily may be seen mixing their white locks with boys, & pursuing their profession with the ardor of youth; there is not a solitary great man in France that is idle,...Witness Broussais lecturing & labouring daily to sustain himself after having elevated himself to the pinnacle - Lisfranc an old bachelor worth thousands, who after making his daily visit for ten mos; from duty, during the vacation of 2 mos: from choice gives a course of operation - and old Rullier may be seen daily supporting himself from bedpost to bedpost, as jolly as if he were not over sixty, & Velpeau born a poor boy without money, time, education, or friends, has by industry made himself one of the first surgeons in Europe - then let no one say he is industrious unless he can show a mountain that he has moved.[20]

Home Again

Bassett returned to Huntsville and built a successful practice. As might be expected from his attention to anatomical dissection and the mentors he most respected in Paris - Velpeau and Helmagrand - his practice developed in a destined way. As Mastin noted in his letter to Osler,

> [Bassett's] knowledge of Anatomy and his preferences for surgery gave him the surgical cases of that section of the county and he soon became the recognized surgeon of North Alabama....But he never enjoyed the confidence and respect of the community at large, and chiefly on account of the opposition he met at the hands of his co-workers in the profession.[21]

His enlarging practice was also influenced by the growing awareness, both among his colleagues and the general public, that a man who had studied in England and in France might well know more than physicians trained locally. Consultations and referrals by other physicians improved his professional standing.

His personal reputation in the community was another matter. His spinster sister and his mother moved from Baltimore to Huntsville, apparently making his standing in the community even worse. As Carmichael noted in his article, "Margaret, a woman of education, disappointed hopes and endowed with a liberal share of bitter sarcasm, stirred up strife in the community and John had to bear the brunt of it all."[22] Bassett appears to have consciously chosen positions that ran contrary to many in his community. He seems to have been a very judgmental man, finding faults in most of the established structures in society. As Carmichael noted,

John Young was an unusual character....[H]e was never content with accepting any condition as he found it just because it existed. There was slavery, religion, quackery, and professional stupidity. Sooner or later he would ridicule each of their weaknesses. He outraged the institution of slavery. His friends and associates felt that he did not have the proper reverence for the church and religion because he questioned many of its established rights.[23]

As an owner of slaves Bassett took severe exception to the efforts of a local pastor to work towards its abolition. He wrote numerous articles for local newspapers using a pen name, attacking the efforts of abolitionists in Scotland and Ireland to join the Presbyterian Synod in America in denouncing slavery. Bassett was a complicated person.

Bassett wrote an article for each of the two volumes of Fenner's *Southern Medical Reports* of 1849-50 and 1850-51. Both were on climatic factors and their influences on diseases and their treatments as he tabulated them in Madison County. In his case histories he very carefully described symptoms, prescribed treatments, outcomes, and autopsy findings, when they were done. His treatment routine was that of the heroic style with bleeding, purging, emetics, cold water applications, quinine and other popular medications. In his 1849-50 article he gave some statistics:

Of the thirty physicians in the county, six reside in Huntsville, and do about twelve thousand dollars worth of good practice. We have also a German Root-Doctor, a Homoeopathist, a Steam Doctor and several negro Faith-Doctors....
There is about ten thousand dollars worth of medicines sold annually in the county (including about 80 pounds of calomel and 1,000 ounces of quinine) of which about $5,000 is quackery,[24]

In 1848 Bassett was instrumental in organizing the Medical Society of Madison County of which he was elected secretary at its first meeting. The call to the organizing meeting, published in the newspaper, *Southern Advocate,* sought "practitioners of medicine of Madison County who are graduates of respectable schools and who have not habitually indulged in quackery,..."[25] There were initially sixteen members.

Bassett's studies of the climate factors thought to be definitive of regional differences in diseases provided him with an outlet for his scientific interests piqued in Paris. He also thought through some of the philosophical questions about the practice of medicine. He recognized that some diseases were self-limited. At the head of his article for the 1850-51 volume of *Southern Medical Reports* he quoted Celsus on treatment: "Celsus thought it better, in doubtful cases, to try a doubtful remedy, than none at all." In his ongoing studies and in his practice Bassett found the opposite to be true. He continued,

> I will, therefore, only say that I have been fortunate, in my own practice, in reversing the aphorism at the head of this article; that rule of practice has found favor in the eyes of every generation of both doctors and patients, and it is not wonderful that the few able men of every age that have opposed it have warred in vain - that the science of French expectancy, and the quackery of German Homoeopathy, have alike failed: dying men will have pills and parsons.[26]

Bassett was a student of Nature. He felt that a student of medicine must have an enduring concern to learn the normal functions of the body if diseases are ever to be understood. He called this study, physiology, the *open sesame* to the profession of medicine, just the beginning of the real work of the physician.

> [H]e will be led to his ultimate object, to take his last lessons from the poor and suffering, the fevered and phrenzied, from the Jobs and Lazaruses - into the pest-houses and prisons, and here, in these magazines of misery and contagion, these Babels of disease and sin, he must not only take up his abode, but following the example of his Divine Master, he must love to dwell there; - this is Pathology.[27]

Commentary

One of the remarkable gifts that William Osler bequeathed to us was his tenacity in pursuit of an event, a person, an idea, or a hint from past or present that might enlighten him - and us. The story of John Y. Bassett is an example of the intellectual curiosity that Osler encouraged in his students and colleagues. Not only was Osler interested in the medical and historical facts about malaria; he found and read the two volumes of an obscure journal published briefly 45 years previously in New Orleans. From this he went on to find out what he could about one the authors, a forgotten physician, the subject of this essay. This type of intellect makes a superb teacher and role model for all generations.

Bassett himself is a figure to admire despite some of his personal characteristics. Apparently he had a sad and tear-filled childhood. He went on to study medicine and practice in a community far removed from home, bedeviled by an angry and tormented sister, and at odds with many of the conventions and beliefs of his time. In pursuit of some undescribed hunger he went to London and Paris in 1835-1836 to learn from the leaders of his profession. His letters inform us of his experiences and impress us with his commitments to his chosen work.

Certainly, for one man - Bassett's apprentice and the author of the letter to Osler - Claudius H. Mastin, M.D., Bassett was unique. He wrote,

> My observation whilst a college student in Virginia had impressed me with the conviction that the outcome of a man depends more, as a general thing, on his first preceptor than on any subsequent instructor, for it is from him that he acquires the mental habitudes which subsequently lead him on to accuracy and distinction or to the looseness and inaccuracy with the necessary failure that these faults involve. The wisdom of my action has been verified by the subsequent history of my life.[28]

At the close of his essay on Bassett, Osler noted that he had shown

> Dr. Bassett to have been a man of more than ordinary gifts, but he was among the voiceless of the profession. Nowadays environment, the opportunity for work, the skirts of happy chance carry men to the summit. To those restless spirits who have had ambition without opportunities, and ideals not realizable in the world in which they move, the story of his life may be a solace.[29]

Bassett developed tuberculosis in 1851. He went to Florida in hope of recovering, returning home in the fall, to die on November 2, 1851 at the age of 46. This brief account of this distant physician may make us wish we could have known him better.

---

[1]Osler, William, "An Alabama Student," *An Alabama Student and Other Biographical Essays,* London, Oxford University Press, 1908, 2.

[2]Osler, Ibid., 2.
[3]Osler, Ibid., 2.
[4]Mastin, Claudius H., "A Letter from Doctor Claudius H. Mastin to Doctor Osler on Incidents in the Life of John Y. Bassett," *The Medical Reports of John Y. Bassett, M.D.,* with Introduction by Daniel C. Elkin, M.D., Charles C. Thomas, 1941, 58.
[5]Carmichael, Emmett B., "John Young Bassett: The Alabama Student," *J. M. A. Alabama,* 34:2, 1964, 31.
[6]Bassett, John Young, Letter to his wife March 27, 1836.
[7]Mastin, *op. cit.,* 59-60.
[8]Mastin, Ibid., 60.
[9]Bassett, Letter to his wife, 1 February 1936.
[10]Ibid.
[11]Ibid., March 11, 1836.
[12]Ibid., March 16, 1836.
[13]Ibid., July 10, 1836.
[14]Ibid., July 3, 1836.
[15]Warner, John Harley, *Against the Spirit of System,* Princeton, Princeton University Press, 1998, 177-178.
[16]Bassett, Letter to his sister, September 5, 1836.
[17]Ibid., April 29, 1836.
[18]Ibid., Letter to his wife, March 13, 1836.
[19]Ibid., March 13, 1836.
[20]Ibid., September 13, 1836.
[21]Mastin, *op. cit.,* 61.
[22]Carmichael, *op. cit.,* 32-33.
[23]Ibid., 33.
[24]Bassett, John Young, T*he Medical Reports of John Y. Bassett, op. cit.,* 5.
[25]Carmichael, *op. cit.,* 33.
[26]Ibid., 44.
[27]Ibid., 47, 49.
[28]Mastin, *op. cit.,* 62.
[29]Osler, *op. cit.,* 18.

Chapter 5

Henry Ingersoll Bowditch, 1808-1892

A study of Henry Ingersoll Bowditch offers a remarkable view of the professional and personal careers of an American physician in the turbulent years of the nineteenth century. He lived in a time of radical change in the social context of the United States, a time when established hallmarks of society - religion, social class, occupation, race, and nationality - were called into question. Bowditch lived in the years that saw the end of the Frontier, and the growth of industrialization as we entered the Gilded Age; Charles Darwin published works that changed forever our view of the created order; the Civil War was a wrenching experience for the entire country; the Transcendentalist Movement - a brief period of brilliant writing and thought - remains a gem in American history; the introduction of anesthesia and the discovery of bacteria leading to a germ theory of disease turned medicine on its head when added to the explosion caused by the clinical and laboratory revolution instigated in Europe. Medicine was redefined and reconstructed.

Bowditch was alert to these changes and his life would be determined by his involvement in them. He confronted the turmoil of his time and defined himself by his work, not merely his words. Abolition of slavery, the liberation of women to vote and work on a par with men, the new field of preventive medicine, and the broad concerns of the Reform Movement - all these merited his committed attention. These issues also caused him to question established moral determinants such as organized religion and politics; he saw in them deterrents to both social and personal growth and enrichment sufficient enough to question his full acceptance of any doctrine. Bowditch lived in a time and a place where these issues were constantly being defined by debate, by literary excellence, and by action; he counted among his close friends the Emersons, John Greenleaf Whittier, James Russell Lowell, Louis Agassiz, Theodore Parker, and the Channings, all persons of courage and conviction, able and willing to witness to their beliefs with both their words and their works.

Bowditch was born in Salem, Massachusetts, the third son of an internationally respected mathematician. Raised in an era of strict

Puritanical religious observances, his parents held more liberal views; they were able to encourage in him a religious sensibility that would inform him for the rest of his life, although he declined to join any church or confess to any creed. The family moved to Boston when he was fifteen; his father accepted the position of Actuary of the Massachusetts Hospital Life Insurance Company. Bowditch attended the Public Latin School and entered Harvard as a sophomore at the age of seventeen in 1825. An interesting side note is that the one regret Bowditch had of the early years of his education was not being allowed to indulge his great love of music, a luxury his father considered a waste of valuable time.

His college years seem to have been quite ordinary, as suggested by an uninteresting diary. One comment, however, displays his imaginative use of language, and offers a lesson to preachers. After listening to a sermon, Bowditch wrote in his diary, "Dr. Ware preached one of his dry sermons. It put me in mind of spinning glass, where out of a little piece they spin several thousand yards."[1]

In a delightful note in his biographical study of his father, Vincent Y. Bowditch wrote,

Previous to his graduation from college in 1828, my father had shown no special taste nor talent which would lead him to choose the practice of medicine for his life work....He felt himself quite unfit for the study of law or the ministry, and the life of a business man was most uncongenial to him. With a feeling of doubt, almost of indifference, not unmixed with repugnance toward some of the elementary work necessary to all who study medicine, he entered Harvard Medical School. He often spoke of his sudden change of feeling when, after the sense of loathing at the idea of "cutting up a dead body," the demonstrator of anatomy showed to him, in a dissection, the wonderful arrangement of the muscles of the forearm. His chief instructor was Dr. James Jackson, a noble man, a wise and conscientious physician and excellent teacher, who in those days stood at the head of his profession in Boston.[2]

This attention to immediate experiences and an alertness to his interior responses to them would be definitive of his personal and his professional development. We have heard of Dr. Jackson before, the physician who took Jacob Bigelow as his partner; we will hear of him again for the crucial role he played in Boston as a model for the ideal physician, clinically, morally, and as a citizen.

The Paris Years

Bowditch was an intern under Jackson after graduating from medical school. In the Spring of 1832 he decided that study in Paris was a necessity, and sailed to Havre. There he would join other doctors who came to pursue new ways of learning medicine at the Paris Clinical School. Among these was his close friend, James Jackson, Jr., the brilliant son of Bowditch's Harvard instructor and perennial professional model; Jackson, Jr. would die of typhoid fever the next year. Bowditch carried with him a letter of introduction from George Ticknor, professor of belle-lettres at Harvard and a leading light in the academic world. The letter was addressed to Alexander von Humboldt, the renowned German geographer who was a frequent visitor to Paris. This letter, accompanying a translation by Bowditch's father of the second volume of *Mecanique Celeste* by the mathematician, La Place, assured the new student of immediate acceptance into the Paris School. Bowditch entered the École de Médecine where he became a student - and subsequently a friend - of Pierre Louis, to whom he was introduced by James Jackson, Jr.

Pierre Louis had a remarkable effect on Bowditch, one that Bowditch outlined in a talk he gave before the Boston Society for Medical Observation in 1872, shortly after the death of Louis. Bowditch studied under Louis for two and a half years, returning to Boston in the Spring of 1835. Commenting on his time in Paris with Louis he said,

> I had had special courses with various individuals; but my chief, I may almost say my only, Parisian medical education had been with him. He had moulded my medical mind into such a rigid belief in the necessity of strict deductions from facts actually studied out with the utmost care at the bedside that, for a time, I flippantly talked about all that had preceded us as if their influence was to be deemed of no importance in the presence of the exceeding light that strict observation was to thrown on medicine....[I]t is astonishing how little of the details of medical diagnosis and prognosis which I learned of him I have found erroneous.[3]

Although Bowditch had important contacts with outstanding men such as the physiologist, Magendie, who invited him to visit on the wards at Hôtel Dieu, it was Louis who was most instructive.

Jackson, Jr. who had been with Louis for nearly two years, left for home, and Bowditch took his place with deep gratitude. He practically took on the position of an *interne,* visiting and examining patients on the wards, attending autopsies, but - most importantly - learning the necessity of careful observation and recording of facts from examination. Bowditch wrote in his diary when he learned of Louis's death, that he "caught some of his keen, rapid, but very truthful methods of observing....I felt at one of his analyses of a new case as if new scenes in medical diagnosis were suddenly opened before me."[4] A fellow American student, Dr. Pierson of Salem, after watching Bowditch at work on the wards, told him, "You probably know more about the diagnosis of disease than any one in Boston." Bowditch wrote, "I, of course, was pleased, but I turned all the credit to my master beloved."[5]

In 1832 Louis was asked by a small group of students to be the president of a new study group, the Society for Medical Observation. The students had three objectives in mind: 1), to learn the methods of careful observation and present the findings to the group; 2), to influence their profession to attend to the importance of accuracy in observation; 3), to publish both their findings and examples of the method of Louis.[6] Two other highly regarded teachers, Andral and Chomel, were honorary presidents of the Society. The learning process was a strict one, painful at times. The students were required to criticize each other at their weekly meetings, which they did, often in ways that tended to show off their own knowledge. Bowditch recalled one evening when, after being put down by two of his fellow students, Louis moved in on him. Bowditch wrote,

> If my compeers had hit hard with their random shots, he would, it seemed annihilate me, as in fact he finally did on one of my points: viz., that because I had not carefully examined *one side of it,* I "might as well have omitted all reference to the subject"! And with this our meeting ended.[7]

Bowditch noted that it was with "grim delight" that he reviewed the evening: it was difficult, but he had learned. The Society had an impact on the students that would persist. Comparable Societies were established in London and in Boston when the students returned home with the purpose of keeping alive the strenuous searching for knowledge that was becoming so important for the new scientific approach to medicine. However, these Societies, lacking the relentless drive for observation that propelled Louis, were tame successors of the original.

The experiences that Bowditch had in Paris, certainly mirrored in the writings of his friends, Jackson, Jr., Holmes, Warren and others, were extraordinary for them all. Bowditch, writing home in 1833, summed up his views.

I shall always love him, and look upon him as one who is to be a renovator of the science of medicine. He marks out a path for himself and his disciples, but if it be followed closely it can't fail of making medicine a little more certain than it is now, and them more powerful in distinguishing diseases.[8]

Central to our understanding of the importance of Louis is thinking through what was called, the Numerical Method. Louis was a collector of data, both by observing patients on the wards and by detailed analysis of data obtained at autopsy. The goal, obviously, was a correlation of these two sets of findings so that one could arrive at 1), a clear picture of the nature of the disease clinically and pathologically, and 2), a method of analyzing the effectiveness of any specific therapy. There was considerable opposition on both sides of the Atlantic to this Method.

In 1840, Martyn Paine, M.D. published an essay, "On the Principal Writings of P. Ch. A. Louis, M.D.," in a two-volume work, *Medical and Physiological Commentaries.* In this essay he criticized what he labeled 'the Anatomical Method' of medical study. He defended bedside observation as the proper method of establishing a diagnosis, using the appearance of the tongue as one of the major diagnostic tools. He voiced doubts about autopsy findings, suggesting that the effects of 'putrefaction' after death - not the disease - might well explain the findings of the pathologist. He had no objections to tabulating the results of one's findings; he just did not accept the relationships between the bedside and the autopsy findings. The confusion at that time between typhoid and typhus fevers made the argument even more complicated since the classical finding in typhoid fever of damage to the oval elevated areas of lymphoid tissue of the small intestine known as Peyer's patches was not seen in typhus. Another major problem in medicine at that time that concerned many doctors was the rumor that Louis had proven that bloodletting was worthless as a treatment for pneumonia and other diseases. This attack on Louis and his method of study prompted an immediate response from Bowditch.

In three September 1840 issues of *The Boston Medical and Surgical Journal* (later to become *The New England Journal of Medicine)* Bowditch castigated Paine for his discussion of Louis. He made the point that pathology, important as it is, is not the only guide to medical knowledge. He wrote,

We must say that we are devoted lovers of the plan originally proposed by others, but first developed by Louis, viz., the Numerical Method....We look upon pathological anatomy as only one means of deciding the question, and not more important than symptomatology. They stand upon a par; one explains and is connected with the other, and the man who neglects either is a *one-sided* philosopher and will be wholly incapable of any general views.[9]

The widespread rumor that bloodletting was useless as therapy also needed to be modified because it was unbelievable to so many doctors. Since the time of Benjamin Rush it had been the foundation of treatment for any cause of inflammation (fever) and to degrade it was heresy. Actually, Louis waffled a bit on the issue. In the 1836 publication in English of his book, *Researches on the Effects of Bloodletting...,* Louis states

> [W]e infer that bloodletting has had very little influence on the progress of pneumonitis...in the cases under my observation; that its influence has not been more evident in the cases bled copiously and repeatedly, than in those bled only once and to a small amount;...that in cases where it appears to be otherwise, it is undoubtedly owing, either to an error in diagnosis, or to the fact that the bloodletting was practised at an advanced period of the disease,...[10]

He recommended minimal bloodletting at the onset of the disease, finding it of no value later. His basic work, though, known as the Numerical Method was the beginning of the use of statistics to evaluate findings in all areas of science.

Bowditch was impressed by the freedom for education that Paris provided. In writing to his father he looked forward to working in Boston to open the libraries and the museums to the public freely, and not continue the English tradition of making people pay for everything. He obviously had been infected with the excitement of the opportunities for learning in the City of Lights and he hoped to bring that excitement home with him. A brief trip to England confirmed his conviction that the English and Scottish schools had nothing exceptional to offer. He wrote to his father that the physicians talked a lot but seemed to know very little; the heyday of English supremacy was over. His father obviously thought differently and was opposed to his staying in Paris. Bowditch deftly turned his argument to his father by asking, if his father came to Paris to study mathematics with an exciting and earnest teacher, would he want to go to England where the teachers might not know as much as he did already? The argument was over and Bowditch stayed on as a pupil of Louis.

A fascinating aside about the differences between medical education in England and in France is revealed in a pamphlet published in 1828 by William Mackenzie (1791-1868), *Use of the Dead to the Living*. Mackenzie addressed the short supply of bodies for dissection by students; only the bodis of executed criminals could be used. The need for anatomical subjects was critical. He wrote,

> The basis of all medical and surgical knowledge is anatomy. Not a single step can be made either in medicine or surgery, considered either as an art or a science, without it....
> Disease, which is the object of these arts to prevent and to cure, is denoted by disordered function: disordered function cannot be understood without a knowledge of healthy function; healthy function cannot be understood without a knowledge of structure; structure cannot be understood unless it be examined.[11]

Mackenzie continued with a discussion of various diseases and surgical conditions in which anatomical knowledge was important. He concluded with the observations that, 1), any British student who can afford it goes to Paris, 2), schools in England and Scotland will be deserted, and 3), England will become dependent upon France. His solution, logically and clearly stated, was to copy the French and make unclaimed bodies of the deceased available to the medical schools.

Bowditch took some time off and went to Italy in 1834, shortly before coming home. He followed the physicians on their hospital rounds in Genoa.

> [T]he result was that I was glad to have studied in Paris. Each physician has 200 patients. Some he speaks to, others he remains perhaps a minute, but the same indefiniteness of ideas in regard to the disease they are treating is manifested that we meet everywhere else save in the wards of Louis. They all have their theories and act up to them.[12]

When Bowditch was in Milan he received letters from his brother telling of his mother's death. He was terribly upset, grieving, and yet rebellious that he had not been home at that time. He went into the cathedral, and, as he entered the organist began to play. The 'divine' effect of music on him was apparent. His son wrote that,

> The sense of perfect peace which came over him remained with him, and he left the cathedral soothed and comforted. It was a striking illustration of a phase of his character seen often in later life, when, in the midst of crushing sorrow, his spirit seemed to be uplifted and calmed by similar influences in a manner that to many would seem almost incomprehensible.[13]

In 1834 Bowditch returned to Boston, set up his practice and became a leading physician in the city. He subsequently married an English woman, Olivia Yardley, whom he would refer to as "one of the brightest gems of life." His father was quick to 'adopt' her as his second daughter.

Highlights of a Medical Career

On October 21, 1835, one year after Bowditch opened his office, he had another experience that changed the direction of his life. He had left his office and was walking down Washington Street when he encountered a mob of well-dressed men in front of the old State House. He was told that they were there in an effort to get William Lloyd Garrison and George Thompson - two avowed Abolitionists - out of the building and 'tar and feather' them. There was a very strong crusade afoot to stop the anti-slavery movement. Bowditch spoke with a friend who was a city official and who agreed with the need to suppress the Abolitionists. Bowditch wrote in his diary,

> I was completely disgusted, and vowed in my heart as I left him with utter loathing, "I am an Abolitionist from this very moment, and tomorrow I will subscribe for Garrison's 'Liberator.'" I ever after kept my word, and now thank Heaven that among the greatest blessings of my life I can look upon this mob, and my introduction to Garrison in consequence thereof, as two of the choicest events of my existence.[14]

Bowditch remained a dedicated opponent of slavery despite the rejections he suffered from friends and from the social elite in Boston who disagreed strongly with the efforts of the antislavery movement.

In 1835 Bowditch began to work as a volunteer at the Warren Street Chapel, a non-denominational organization that devoted its energies to helping the children of the poor. Bowditch was cheered by the children, but distressed by the formal religious observance he witnessed. As the nation moved steadily toward a bitter confrontation with slavery, ministers and priests attempted to provide biblical proof of its acceptance by God. Another example that concerned him was that, as alcoholism seemed to be spreading, particularly among the poor, the blame was being placed upon the drunkard, absolving those whom he saw encouraging drinking. The religious organizations seemed utterly committed to maintaining the *status quo*. Bowditch spoke to the children about slavery and even attempted to bring some 'colored' children into the Chapel program. This was a turning point;

his suggestions were dismissed as impossible and he discontinued his relationship with the program that had been so meaningful for him.

Bowditch constantly attempted to hold his understanding of a moral and religious life in harmony with his position as a physician. Soon after beginning his practice he was appointed admitting physician to the Massachusetts General Hospital (MGH). In 1841, at a time of serious and often vicious confrontations between Abolitionists and pro-slavery groups, the trustees of the hospital voted to exclude 'colored people' from the hospital. Bowditch promptly submitted his resignation from the staff; the trustees reconsidered their decision, and the resignation was not accepted. His association with MGH continued for decades thereafter.

In 1846 Bowditch formed the Society for Medical Observation closely modeled on the original Paris group. The Society, originally composed of twelve doctors, including instructors at the medical school, met twice a month to discuss medical papers. Although Bowditch attempted to keep the group in the same style as the Paris one, apparently the criticisms were harsh enough that some members resigned. In 1859, at the age of 51, he was appointed Jackson Professor of Clinical Medicine at Harvard, a position he held until he resigned in 1867 to devote his energies to other causes.

An impressive achievement of Bowditch was promoting the use of the procedure called thoracentesis: puncturing the chest with a needle to drain pus or other liquid from the pleural space. Untreatable lung diseases such as pneumonia and tuberculosis, and injuries to the chest that caused internal bleeding were causes of pleural effusion, the most prominent symptom of which was shortness of breath. Most doctors hoped - and said - that the fluid would go away with time, but this rarely happened. Occasional efforts were made in Europe to insert a trochar by 1840. In 1844 two English doctors published, in the *Guy Hospital Reports,* their experiences with successfully treated cases by use of a surgical incision; this report encouraged Bowditch to inquire further. When he asked the opinion of the procedure of a renowned Philadelphia auscultator, he was told, "I would as soon send a bullet into the chest as plunge a trochar into it."[15] Bowditch persisted in his interest and was delighted to find a Doctor Wyman in Cambridge, Massachusetts who did the procedure and had appropriate equipment for it. Under the instruction of Wyman, Bowditch did his first thoracentesis in 1850, and it was a success. From 1850 to 1870 he did a total of 250 tappings on 154 persons with no fatalities. It is important to recall that there were really no methods of treating this condition and no antibiotics to treat the infections commonly associated with it.

Bowditch listed his reasons for doing the procedure, and they included saving life, prolonging life by giving temporary relief, and treating early rather than waiting for worsening of the condition. As we might expect, there were physicians in England and France who accepted thoracentesis immediately; most doctors there and in the United States rejected it; the Viennese sneered at it. Bowditch was quick to stress that this procedure was not to be used as a last resource for patients, but applied early when there was hope for success. An important part of this anecdote is that Bowditch, although often credited with the institution of the procedure, always referred to other physicians who had preceded him. It was his style to always give credit to others for ideas and for actions. He went to Europe in 1859 to present his findings.

During his stint in Paris in the 1830s Bowditch became very adept at auscultation under the tutelage of Louis. He continued his interest in diseases of the heart and lungs and in 1846 published a guide for medical students, *The Young Stethoscopist.* Dedicated to James Jackson, Sr., his mentor in years past, it is a remarkable text that includes listening to the head, to the larynx, to arteries and veins, and to animals. It was a good text for students of that time; the clinical wisdom of Bowditch for that era - and for ours - is revealed in his introduction. He wrote,

> For you I have prepared this book on physical diagnosis....Its name indicates its object; viz.: to give you, in a compact form, a complete view of what are technically called the physical signs. But I have another, and perhaps equally important end in view, viz.: to make you feel that the *time,* the *place,* the *circumstances* in which you may meet with these morbid signs, and the relations which they bear to the rational signs, are of as much importance as the physical signs themselves.[16]

By the 1850s Bowditch restricted his practice to diseases of the heart and lungs. His skills in auscultation and in thoracentesis placed him in the position of a consultant on diseases of the chest in New England. Bowditch was also a major performer of autopsies at MGH, following the example of his mentor, Louis.

Interest in pulmonary diseases led him to a study of the incidence of tuberculosis - known popularly as consumption - in Massachusetts. There were competing theories of the cause of this devastating disease, and Bowditch surveyed the state, town by town, to determine the local incidence and the residences of the patients. He was convinced that damp soil was instrumental in causing what was also called, phthisis (or phthysis). In an amazing booklet, *Consumption in New England:*

or, Locality One of its Chief Causes, published in 1862, Bowditch correlated location of patients with humidity of soil and air, confirming for him that these factors were instrumental in the cause of the disease, coming down, finally, to calling it a law. It is interesting that in an address to The Boston Society for Medical Observation two years later, his position had changed slightly. His final statement in the paper was,

First. - Consumption is not *contagious* in the usual acceptance of that word.
Second. - It may be *infectious*, and to this extent only. By long attendance of the closest kind, by inhaling the breath of the phthisical patient, by living in the phthisical atmosphere, so to speak, and in general by a neglect of hygienic laws during such attendance, the health may be undermined and phthisis set in.[17]

These studies were in the days before Robert Koch discovered the tubercle bacillus; we may smile at them, but still attend to the efforts some made to understand the diseases their patients presented to them.

A delightful and revealing side note about Bowditch relates to his search for a sun dial in 1846 to place in front of a small country house he bought in Weston. He heard that Dr. Waterhouse, a member of the first faculty at the medical school who had recently died, had brought a sun dial with him from England. Bowditch was given the dial by one of Waterhouse's descendents; he then requested his friend, John Greenleaf Whittier, to write a few lines to put on the face of the dial. Whittier complied, sending the following lines:

With warning hand I mark Time's rapid flight
From life's glad morning to its solemn night;
Yet, through the dear God's love I also show
There's light above me by the shade below.[18]

Engraved on a brass plate with the signs of the Zodiac, the dial was a treasure for Bowditch.

The passage of the Fugitive Slave Law in 1850 intensified the drive of the Abolitionists for ending slavery; bounty hunters appeared in northern cities and demanded that public authorities assist them in finding and returning slaves who had fled the South. Bowditch joined with those who protected fugitives from capture. An Anti-Man-Hunting League was formed in 1854. The elaborate plan called for an immediate assembling of the members of the League if, and when, a fugitive hunter appeared so that his efforts could be blocked and the fugitive protected. To many it seemed an odd, even grotesque response to the situation, but feelings ran high and the capture of an escaped slave and his return to the South was considered an abomination. The League did little except keep their strong opposition to the federal law prominently displayed. An important result of the passage of the law was the downfall of Daniel Webster, a famous senator who made the grave error of voting for the law in exchange for possible support in his bid for presidential nomination. The writings about Webster that evolved confirmed the near disbelief of the people that he would do this. Vincent Y. Bowditch, commenting on his father's response, wrote,

> Up to the very last days of his life my father spoke in no measured terms of what he deemed the perfidy of Daniel Webster, who, at the last hour...suddenly astounded and disappointed all those who were anxiously awaiting the effect of his words in Congress by telling the North that "they must conquer their prejudices" and accept the measure. From that time forward, no argument or excuse could convince my father that Webster had done other than prostitute his "God-like intellect" for sordid ends.[19]

The beginning of the Civil War was a time of crisis in the United States. The Army was unprepared for the staggering medical demands it faced. The need for physicians and surgeons to care for the huge number of men wounded or plagued with dysentery, the lack of hospital facilities, a non-existent ambulance corps, and the general ineptitude of governmental services overwhelmed all efforts to care for the armies. As noted before, the level of education and training of most physicians was particularly lacking in the skills needed on the battlefield or in the camps. In 1862 Bowditch responded to the call of the Governor and volunteered to serve as a physician in Virginia. What appalled him there - aside from the horrors of the battles - was the absence of any ambulance services. There were wagons driven by men with no training that carried the wounded and dying away from the field; Bowditch was horrified to note that the driver of his wagon was drunk. Bowditch went to great efforts to get Congress to form an ambulance corps. His efforts on behalf of the soldiers was greatly influenced by the death of his eldest son in the battle of Potomac Creek in March 1863. He translated his grief into renewed correspondence and political pressure on the Congress to provide such an elementary service for the Army. He finally achieved that goal in 1863, and considered it one of his major accomplishments.

Vincent, a younger son of Bowditch and author and editor of his biography, noted that there was a beautiful yet tragic pathos resting upon that part of what may be justly called the stirring drama of my father's life, in its connection with the great anti-slavery movement and the death of my brother, when we call to mind the incident of the little boy of eleven taken from his bed in the early morning by his father to witness the return of the slave to a life of bondage, and when we ponder upon the significance of that act to both father and son.[20]

The interest that Bowditch had in tuberculosis spurred his commitment to preventive medicine and the public health. Beginning in 1866 there was pressure from prominent citizens on the Massachusetts House of Representatives to create a state board of health. This was accomplished in 1869 when the Governor appointed seven men: three physicians, one lawyer, one civil engineer, a business man and an historian to the Board. Bowditch was elected chair of the committee and remained active on it for ten years. One of Bowditch's insights into the role of preventive medicine was laid out by him in the Fifth Annual Report of the State Board of Health. He presented a series of recommendations that, as he wrote, "any experienced physician might even now give according to the principles and rules of actions that will weigh with the physicians of the future." He continued,

I believe that if these recommendations, with others that might be added by any family physician, should be thoroughly carried out by the parent during childhood...many that would otherwise possibly have died of consumption will escape that calamity....I contend therefore that the physician of the future will stand higher than ever as preventive medicine advances.[21]

In 1878 the Governor merged three boards - health, lunacy, and charity - to create a chaos in which politicians and lawyers struggled for control and advantage. Bowditch resigned in 1879, the same year in which he was appointed to the National Board of Health, just enacted by Congress. His work there continued to be devoted to preventive medicine, but it encountered the same political roadblocks that he had known at home. He resigned in 1883, in part for reasons of health.

At the September 1876 meeting of the International Medical Congress in Philadelphia Bowditch delivered the Centennial Address. In this lengthy talk he presented a detailed history of the emergence of state public health boards and their importance for preventive medicine. He also made an instructive division of the preceding 100 years into three segments: 1), 1776 to 1832 - the era of Rush and

Broussais; 2) 1832 to 1869 - the era of Louis and the creation of the first state board of health; and 3), 1869 to the future when progress and prevention would produce marked improvements in the health of the nation. This talk was important in that his surveys of Massachusetts and his knowledge and expertise in public health were documented and sent to all the states for their education and possible political enactment. One of the results of this speech was his election, the following year, to the presidency of the American Medical Association.

As the Reform Movement accelerated in the last quarter of the nineteenth century, temperance became a major concern of reformers. There was a strong movement afoot for legal prohibition, for banning the evils of alcohol use - the 'demon rum.' Bowditch supported the idea of temperance but opposed prohibition as the way to alleviate the social problems associated with alcohol abuse. In a way quite characteristic of his method of working, he corresponded with a large number of persons, physicians and laymen in the United States and Europe, asking them to respond to his series of questions. He surveyed the impressions they had about the relationships between habits and behavior: could they relate drinking light wines, beer, and liquors with the levels of drunkenness they saw? The replies he received confirmed his belief that it was liquor that was the problem. Drinking light wines and beer was reported to produce little drunkenness. From this experience he remained a supporter of temperance, convinced that the cure for intemperance lay with moral education, not prohibition by legislative action.

Bowditch was a strong advocate for the right of women to join the American Medical Association, as he was, also, for their admission to the Massachusetts Medical Society. In 1881 he published an article in the *Boston Medical and Surgical Journal* about the hostile attitude of Harvard and the Society toward women. He took a strong civil rights position in the argument to admit women, pointing out the moral error in taking and enjoying for yourself what you deny to others; he also suggested that prohibiting women from becoming well-trained physicians would merely send them elsewhere for education, or perhaps even into quackery. It would take another three years before women would be admitted into the Society and another eighty years before they would be admitted to Harvard Medical School.

Back in 1846, through his work with children in the Warren Chapel, Bowditch became concerned about the lives of tenement dwellers: the effects of poverty on this marginal population. A committee was formed, but not much was done until much later when, in 1870 on a trip to London, he met with a Miss Octavia Hill and Sir Sidney

Waterlow who had each developed new housing projects for the poor. Not only were there new homes, but there were flowers growing in the windows; Bowditch walked through the developments, talking with the tenants who were pleased with their good luck. Surprisingly, the projects were financially stable. On his return to Boston he reported his findings to the State Board of Health, and, more importantly, helped form a corporation with funding that would renovate one of the eyesores of Boston, a three-story tenement known by the name, Crystal Palace. The tenants represented the worst of society in the committee's eyes: non-working drunks, dirty and ragged children, loose women. The building was renovated, a grog shop closed, an industrial school for the children was founded, and the School Street Five Cents Savings Bank accepted accounts of the children's pennies. Although not a great financial success, the Lincoln Building, as it was renamed, spoke to the mature philanthropic efforts of its renovators.

Moral and Religious Issues

Bowditch ordered his life, in both its private and public sectors, by careful analyses of the moral implications of his motives as well as his actions. He seems to the viewer to have stood usually slightly tangential to accepted doctrines and codes, being careful to assess with honesty both his goals and his means of reaching them. Living, as he did, in the years of the blooming of American Transcendentalism, he was strongly influenced by persons such as his friend, Ralph Waldo Emerson, the icon of that philosophy, and the poet, John Greenleaf Whittier, a powerful force in the Abolition Movement. The former was a non-church moralist, the latter a devout Quaker. Both of these men were writers whose lives as well as their works were strong influences on the moral questions of the day. Bowditch attended a number of churches, but was not a member of any one. He sought always to associate with women and men whose actions - political and personal - reflected their professions of faith, whatever they might be.

In an address before the American Academy of Medicine in 1888 Bowditch spoke to the contentious issue of codes of medical ethics, a concern that split the medical profession and sparked arguments and dissension for forty years. He spoke to the two moral forces - tolerance and intolerance - that he found relevant to the profession. He pointed to the lack of clear defining characteristics of these two moral categories, dependent as they are on causation, consequences, and commitments. He spoke to a history of medicine of men such as

Jenner and Harvey who were condemned for their beliefs - understandings that later became foundations of medical science. Bowditch had serious reservations about any 'code' of ethics that would be applicable to all situations, considering the vagaries of experience and of faith. His proposal to the Academy was in three parts. He wrote,

> 1. Let us tolerate any foolish (as we think) or extravagant opinion until at least we have fairly considered it in all its bearings....Let, therefore, tolerance be the rule;...
> 2. No general rules can, I think, safely be laid down that will not, under the influence of passion and bigotry, be liable to do more harm than good....[22]

His third question was, which code should be adopted? His answer reverted back to that ancient moral rule coming out of the dawn of our civilization: we should do to others as we would have them do to us. Bowditch could accept these words as all that would be needed.

Bowditch held firmly to his conviction that each person must think through the relations among faith, action, and community so that moral behavior would be a natural result of reflection and promise. As early as the age of 27 he had thought through these relations and, in a remarkable letter to a minister in Boston he wrote,

> I take Jesus for my model, and believe it to be my duty to imitate Him and excite others to do so....I bow to no man. I sign no creeds....[M]ethinks we should act upon the principle of the gospel, and not think we are Christians because we go to church. I am neither Unitarian nor Trinitarian, but I strive to be a follower of Christ.[23]

Bowditch spoke of the "Sabbath of his heart," his own time of centering his thoughts upon the relations in his life between faith and action. He studied his interior self, examining what he referred to as the "great periods of life." These are the times of change: new promises, new experiences that inform the heart and mind, and renewed commitments that defined him to himself, to his profession, to his community, and to his God.

Commentary

Bowditch is an exemplar for all, especially for physicians and students. An outstanding aspect of his character is his persistent alertness to the social situation in which he found himself. Beginning with his realization of his need to study at the Paris School, he appears to have persistently observed his own development as a spouse and a parent, as a member of society, as a responsible citizen, and as a man with an inner religious faith that he sought to show forth with his life. At the same time, he closely observed the stupendous social phenomena of his years: slavery, the plight of the poor, the Civil War, radical changes taking place in American medicine (therapeutics, medical organizations, ethical codes, women's rights, racial policies, public health issues), and the role of government in supervising the health of the nation. He was quick to give credit to others for advances in medicine and in corrections of social disorders. His interests in medicine included preventive health concerns, newer methods of diagnosis and treatment, and bonding the profession together in political, moral, and intellectual ways that would ensure a healthier nation.

[1]Bowditch, Vincent Y., *Life and Correspondence of Henry Ingersoll Bowditch*, Boston and New York, Houghton, Mifflin and Company, 1902, vol. I, 13.
[2]Ibid., 13-14.
[3]Bowditch, Henry I., *Brief Memories of Louis and Some of his Contemporaries*, Boston, Press of John Wilson and Son, 1872, 30-31.
[4]Bowditch, V.Y., *Life...*, op.cit., vol. II, 271.
[5]Ibid., 273.
[6]Bowditch, H.I., *Brief Memories..., op.cit.,* 11-12.
[7]Ibid., 15.
[8]Bowditch, V.Y., *Life..., op. cit.,* vol. I, 38.
[9]H.I.B., (Bowditch, Henry I.), *The Boston Medical and Surgical Journal,* XXIII: No. 5, September 9, 1840, 78.
[10]Louis, P. CH. A., *Researches on the Effects of Bloodletting...,* translated by C.G. Putnam, M.D., Boston, Hilliard, Gray, & Company, 1836, 22.
[11]Mackenzie, William, *Use of the Dead to the Living,* London, Baldwin and Crodock, 1828, 3-4.
[12]Bowditch, Vincent Y., *op. cit.,* I, 75.
[13]Ibid., 80.
[14]Ibid., 100.
[15]Bowditch, Henry I., *Thoracentesis,* New York, William Wood & Co., 1870, 4.
[16]Bowditch, Henry I., *The Young Stethoscopist,* Boston, William D. Ticknor & Co., 1846, v.
[17]Bowditch, Henry I., *Is Consumption Ever Contagious, or Communicated by One Person to Another in Any Manner?,* Boston, David Clapp, 1864, 13.
[18]Bowditch, Vincent Y., *Life..., op. cit.,* I, 245.
[19]Ibid., I, 202.

[20]Ibid., II, 22-23.
[21]Ibid., 234.
[22]Ibid., 256.
[23]Ibid., I, 105.

Chapter 6

John Hoskins Griscom, 1809-1874

In his Preface to his 1972 doctoral thesis on John H. Griscom and the public health of New York, Duncan R. Jamieson wrote,

> If it is true that the strength of a state rests with its people, then all those conditions which significantly affect the people are of importance and of consequence to the historian. Within this context, the steadily deteriorating condition of the public's health in mid-nineteenth century New York City is of more that passing interest to the historian concerned with America's cities, their health, and the intellectual attitudes of the day.[1]

John H. Griscom was a physician in New York City. He had a family medicine practice from 1837 until 1870. He was a respected member of society and was appointed a physician at the New York Dispensary and at the New York Hospital. He is best known to historians of medicine and public health as an unrelenting advocate of improvement in the environment in which the poor lived. Massive immigration in the 1840s, sparked in part by the famine in Ireland, created tenements and labor conditions that made life in New York a close approximation of Hell for the poor. Mortality statistics were alarming and the efforts of the city to provide water, refuse disposal, and livable housing were, to all purposes, insignificant. Decades before the impressive moves for reform that started in the 1850s and 1860s, and long before physicians showed any interest in the health of the poor, Griscom began the work of his lifetime.

What is known about the origins of his commitments to the poor is inferred by his being his father's son. The elder Griscom was a Quaker philanthropist and educator who had an intense interest in the new sciences, especially chemistry, a subject that he made every effort to popularize and introduce to young students. The Quaker influence was prominent in the home, and exposure to the significance of societal conditions for the health of that society was definitive of the work that his son, John H. Griscom would do. Both men were closely allied to those of other religious faiths who also held concerns for the poor central to their lives. Both were collectors of detailed data about the social crises in New York City. The faith of the Society of Friends was central to their self-definition.

H. Richard Niebuhr, in his 1937 landmark book, *The Kingdom of God in America,* commented on the Quaker acceptance of the presence of the kingdom of God in the present time, and its influence on behavior.

> [T]he Quaker was a perfectionist in his social and individual ethics, for he now lived in the new world of God;...Yet he discovered that the kingdom of Christ was by no means the coming kingdom. In fact, if not in theory, he lived in an interim in which he needed to make constant adjustments to an unredeemed world and to abandon his perfectionism.[2]

Griscom was an inheritor of a powerful Quaker expectation of the peaceful revolution that spiritual awakening would bring, yet he had to live as a physician in a world that was glaringly imperfect. Niebuhr, pointing to the writings of one of the premier American Quakers, John Woolman, wrote,

> The revolution Woolman looked for was an individual event taking place in human souls. But the results which he expected were social - the freeing of slaves, the reduction of economic desire, the elimination of poverty through the decrease of wealth which requires poverty for its support, the cessation of war and the establishment of harmony among men.[3]

Reared, as Griscom was, in a religious and philosophical environment that situated the welfare of all persons as an essential human concern, his life and his career offer remarkable examples of commitment to personal faith. The influence of the father on the son - both in religious faith and in the importance of scientific knowledge - is seen in a comment in the Memoir of the elder Griscom.

> [I]t seems to me almost an axiomatic truth, that sound learning and science do, by a natural law, gravitate towards virtue....*Faith in Christ,* when fully admitted as an inmate of the soul, is never satisfied with a merely formal, outward profession of Christ. Its genuine possession is inseparable from the "FRUITS OF THE SPIRIT."[4]

As an interesting aside, it is of note that we know almost nothing of the private, of the social, or of the medical practice segments of the life of his son, the physician.

Education, Training, and Early Career

Griscom attended the New York High School, a private school founded and owned by his father. During a year that his father was abroad, he completed his classical education at his uncle's school in New Jersey, graduating in 1827. Griscom then went to Rutgers Medical College for the prescribed two courses of lectures. He apprenticed in the offices of Dr. John D. Godman, professor of anatomy at Rutgers, and Dr. Valentine Mott, professor of surgery and a leading New York surgeon. The medical school closed, and Griscom completed his medical education at Pennsylvania, the leading medical school in the country. He took two full courses of lectures, wrote his thesis on a diuretic drug for dropsy (subsequently published in the *American Journal of the Medical Sciences,*) and graduated in 1832. He remained as a resident physician for six months and returned to New York to open his office. In 1835 he married Henrietta Peale, a daughter of the painter, Rembrandt Peale; they had eight children. In a biographical sketch written by Samuel W. Francis for the *Medical and Surgical Reporter* in 1866, we read,

> After waiting patiently for sudden cases for the period of three years, the doctor purchased the "good-will" of a physician in the Seventh Ward, who was about to retire, and from that time his circumstances promised remunerative comfort and brought him into immediate contact with a respectable family practice.[5]

Griscom continued to practice until 1870.

In 1833 Griscom became assistant physician at the New York Dispensary and was promoted to physician the following year. In 1834 he began a popular public lecture series on natural philosophy and chemistry that continued for several years. In 1836 he was appointed professor of chemistry at the College of Pharmacy in New York, a position he resigned in 1838. Following in his father's footsteps, Griscom maintained an active interest in chemistry and in physiology, publishing a text, *Animal Mechanism and Physiology,* in 1839, and a very popular school textbook, *First Lessons in Human Physiology,* in 1845. The sixth edition of this text was published in 1847. In his Preface to this work, the influence of his Quaker training appears as Griscom reminded his readers that "anatomy commends itself forcibly to the intelligent mind, as presenting some of the most striking evidences of the wisdom and ingenuity of the Maker of all things.." He claimed that its study will "demonstrate a Supreme Maker and Governor of the Universe."[6] In part associated with the growing importance of chemistry was a fascination with the new discipline of physiology and its valued instruction for the health of the public. This interest would soon be tied to the evolving concerns for the health of the poor that were surfacing in England.

The central figure in the new Sanitary Movement was an English barrister, Edwin Chadwick. Educated in law, he became interested in statistics as related to diseases and deaths in England. He served as Secretary to the New Poor-Law Board starting in 1834; an outbreak of an epidemic in East London in 1838 spurred his interest in legalizing registrations of births and deaths and the causes of the deaths. Sanitation became a central issue for those inquiring into the epidemic and its importance mushroomed. Water supplies, waste disposal, housing, and all related topics became foci of public and governmental concern. Benjamin Ward Richardson, in his "Biographical Dissertation" that is the introduction to a 1887 collection of the writings of Chadwick, wrote,

> [T]he secret of the sanitary idea and the essence of it lay in the conception that the life of man is so influenced and affected by its surroundings, that by a perfected sanitary code the death-rates may be made, practically, whatever we like to make them until we arrive at that natural duration of human existence which is bounded by anatomical and physiological law.[7]

A detailed study of mortality, interment practices, housing, and health was made over several years and, in 1842, the now renowned *Report on the Sanitary Condition of the Labouring Classes of Great Britain* was published; it was written by Chadwick, some 457 pages in length, a triumph for the health of the public. This work would be the model for Griscom.

Another major figure in the Sanitary Movement in England who used the new science of physiology as a tool to educate the public about the relationships between the environment and health was Southwood Smith. His 1835 textbook, *Physiology of Health,* was popular and appeared in some eleven editions. His grandson, G. H., commented in his Preface to the eleventh (revised) 1865 edition that there had been no previous revisions of the book because

> In the course of his practice as a physician, he saw so much disease and misery arising from the neglected state of those districts where the masses of the people are congregated, that he could no longer rest in the vain effort to stem the tide of the evil by medicine; he turned rather to the work of prevention, by purifying the fountain-heads of corruption and infection, and thus became a leader in the small band of pioneers who first roused the country and the Legislature to the necessity of Sanitary Reform.[8]

Conditions of the Laboring Class_

In 1842 Griscom was appointed City Inspector by the Common Council of New York, a position that placed him at the head of the City Health Department. He found himself in charge of a health department in which almost no employee had any medical knowledge or experience. Health Wardens - poorly paid inspectors of public health complaints and problems - rarely fulfilled their duties, terrified as they were to go near sick people, and without training in investigation. Griscom's work in the year of 1842-1843 gave him insight into the living conditions of the poor that provided the impetus for his powerful and effective efforts at reform. He was appointed City Inspector in 1842. John Duffy, in his 1968 book, *A History of Public Health in New York City 1625-1866,* noted that this was

> a step which many municipal officials must have regretted....His report for the year 1842 was a landmark in New York public health. Whereas Dr. Walter's report for the preceding year had contained only three pages of "Remarks," briefly commenting upon the year's statistics, Griscom's report contained an extensive section on mortality statistics...and some 55 pages of commentary....Griscom clearly set forth the thesis that preventive action was a major aim of public health.[9]

Griscom submitted a letter to the mayor at the end of his one year as Inspector. His letter expressed deep concerns for the welfare of the poor and contained suggestions for reform and correction that were profound. The mayor forwarded the letter to a committee: it was rejected. Changes in the political climate closed out any further work he would do for the city at that time.

Griscom, adding some more details to the letter, presented his study as a public address in December 1844, and published it as a pamphlet, *The Sanitary Condition Of the Laboring Population Of New York,* in 1845. The title of his pamphlet is a clear statement of its source in Chadwick's monumental work. Also, in his *A Supplementary Report on the Results of a Spiecal* (sic) *Inquiry...*Chadwick noted his receipt of both of Griscom's reports, *The Sanitary Condition of the Laboring Population of New York* and the Annual Report to the Common Council in 1842. There was mutual interest and influence. Griscom opened his 1845 study with these words, so clearly showing forth his pietistic foundation and his medical training.

> No duty can engage the attention of the magistracy of a city or state, more dignified in itself, more beneficial to the present generation, or more likely

to prove useful to their descendents, than that of procuring and maintaining a sound state of the public health.

Of the three objects contemplated in the Declaration of Independence as necessary to be secured by government, the first named is "Life." Higher purposes cannot be conceived for which governments should be instituted.[10]

Griscom stated his purpose very clearly in capital letters: SANITARY REFORM. And to urge his case he stated the objects of his letter: 1), to demonstrate the high rates of disease, disability, and early death among the poor; 2), to show that these findings are the result of preventable causes; 3), to document that physical evils produce moral evils that are a drain on the financial resources of the city; 4), to detail the means for correcting these evils and preventing their recurrence. Griscom, in establishing the base for his argument for reform, pointed out the impressive differences in mortality statistics between rural and urban dwellers, and between the rich and the poor, further evidence for the need for registration of birth and death statistics.

In those earliest years of the Reform Movement Griscom stressed the essential part that education must play in alleviating the abominations of tenement life.   After an extended discussion of life in the unbelievable horrors of the slums, and the roles that a Health Police (he would prefer *Health Missionaries*) could perform in making things better, Griscom pointed out the central role that education could play in improvement of the health of all classes. Ignorance of what he called 'the laws of life and health' was responsible for much of the injury so apparent among the poor. But, Griscom noted,

> as these evils are not confined to the laboring and destitute part of our population, but also afflict the wealthier portion, a more healthy state of public opinion is absolutely necessary,...
> *This can best, if not only, be done, by making Physiology, as applied to the laws of life, and the prevention of diseases, a subject of study in all our private, public, and common schools.* The children...are the individuals by and with whom, the important change of opinon and habit, is to be wrought, if at all.[11]

In his concluding remarks on the importance of education and of major revisions of the uses of public monies for improvement of the health of all, Griscom commented that the rich, in their well-ventilated and commodious houses, well-fed and well-clothed, need little aid.

They may turn night into day, and dissipate their time and strength in debauchery and folly, but they are not compelled to reside in cellars, and chambers ill-ventilated, or to associate with filth, in foul air. *They* are to be reached only by *moral* teaching.

Griscom wrote that it was those who live in poverty and ignorance

for whom humanity demands that we should employ every means in our power for bettering their physical, as well as their moral, condition.12

Griscom paid close attention to statistical studies from abroad, and noted that the work of Chadwick in London and Du Chatelet in Paris was of crucial importance for this country. The enthusiasm, the talent, and the learning of these men impressed Griscom. He wrote,

It is the cause of Humanity, of the poor, the destitute, the degraded, of the virtuous made vicious by the force of circumstances, which they are now investigating, and exposing to the knowledge of others.[13]

The value of statistics became increasingly obvious and the extensive reports from England were studied with care. Chadwick was an excellent source. Griscom quoted figures from the 1842 *Report on the Sanitary Condition of the Labouring Population of Great Britain* to show that the life expectancy of mechanics, servants, and laborers was between 1/3 and 1/2 of that of professional persons. In Liverpool, for instance, the average age at death of gentry was 35 years, of tradesmen, 22, and of laborers, 15. Another British statistic that impressed Griscom was the difference between age of death in the city as compared to the country, again by class. In Manchester gentry lived 38 years, in Rutlandshire, 52; laborers and mechanics in Manchester lived 17 years, in Rutlandshire, 38. These figures confirmed for Griscom, as they did for Chadwick, that both class and locale were determinative of life expectancy.

Why was this so? Griscom identified the dwelling place of persons as defining their health. The tenement was the scourge of the poor, and for a variety of reasons.

1. Exploitation of poor - often immigrant - laborers by sub-landlords was common. The sub-landlord, not owning the building, disregarded structural and sanitary needs of tenants. Rent was collected in advance and often week by week. Families moved frequently, leaving their trash behind, setting up a pattern of increasing filth in all categories.

2. The construction of the tenements practically eliminated access to fresh air. Windows were a rarity and the possibility of air traveling

from windows to open doors was slight. Clean air was an important, indeed defining, factor for health according to sanitarians of the time.

3. Water was not available in most tenements, and had to be carried in from the street. The impact of this on washing and cleaning in a fifth-floor room was impressive. There were no facilities for either bathing or washing clothes.

4. In immediate proximity with the tenements were horse stables, pig sties, tanneries, gas works, and the slaughter houses that provided meat for the city. There were no available means for disposing of offal and of the waste products that resulted from these works.

5. It was the cellar apartments that most troubled Griscom. He wrote,

> It is almost impossible, when contemplating the circumstances and conditions of the poor beings who inhabit these holes, to maintain the proper degree of calmness requisite for a thorough inspection,...You must descend to them; you must feel the blast of foul air as it meets your face on opening the door; you must grope in the dark, or hesitate until your eye becomes accustomed to the gloomy place,...you must inhale the suffocating vapor of the sitting and sleeping rooms; and in the dark, damp recess, endeavor to find the inmates by the sound of their voices,...all this, and much more, beyond the reach of my pen, must be felt and seen, ere you can appreciate in its full force the mournful and disgusting condition, in which many thousands of the subjects of our government pass their lives.[14]

Griscom was continuing the type of work that his father initiated many years before. In 1817, at a meeting at New York Hospital, the Society for the Prevention of Pauperism was founded, with John Griscom as chairman. The goals included education, job training, temperance work, elimination of begging, and the promotion of savings banks and life insurance. Some six years later a House of Refuge was created by the Society with the statement, "*Resolved,* That it is highly expedient that an institution be formed in this city for promoting the reformation of juvenile offenders, by the establishment of a House of Refuge, for vagrant and depraved young people.[15] Another organization was formed: the Society for the Reformation of Juvenile Delinquents was created to carry out the work. John Griscom was elected a vice-president in 1824.

The distressing fact for his son, John H. Griscom, was that he found the same deplorable conditions in schools, in the City Prison, and in the House of Refuge that his father had founded years before. Another observer, Charles Dickens, reporting on his visit to New York in his 1842 book, *American Notes for General Circulation,* noted

There are many bye-streets, almost as neutral in clean colors, and positive in dirty ones, as bye-streets in London; and there is one quarter, commonly called the Five Points, which, in respect of filth and wretchedness, may be safely backed against Seven Dials, or any other part of famed St. Gile's.[16]

As a result of his findings, Griscom had two questions to place before the magistrate: 1), what are the effects of this style of living on the health of the people and the length of their lives, and 2), what is the effect on their morals, their virtue and their feelings of self-respect? To the first question, Griscom pointed out that, in a city of some 700,000 persons, the dispensaries provided free care to at least 53,000 patient visits in one year, not to mention free care given by private practitioners. Living in squalid conditions and breathing bad air were extremely detrimental to health. It is important to recall that, in the years before Pasteur and Koch, bad air was considered to be the cause, or at least the bearer of, diseases such as cholera, consumption, and many fevers prevalent in the summer months. Not only dispensary visits but causes of death were related to living conditions. About half of the deaths from consumption were in foreigners; three-quarters of dispensary visits were made by natives of other countries, or their children. Griscom wrote,

we are confirmed in the conclusion that the domiciliary condition of these poor beings, the confined spaces in which they dwell, the unwholesome air they breathe, and their filth and degradation are prolific sources of an immense amount of distress and sickness, which in their turn, serve, by the loss of time, of wages, and of strength, to aggravate the miserableness of their condition, to increase the danger to the public health, and the burden of public and private charity.[17]

To the second question about the impact of tenement dwelling on virtue and morality, Griscom was quick to point out that whatever the effects of their style of living, it is the government - i.e., the citizens of the city - who bear the responsibility for the damage done. The passions that all men know are, or can be, held in check by the restrictions of home, workplace, and public areas that we establish. If a family is confined to one room where all human acts - dressing, sleeping, eating, privy use, sexual intercourse - are carried out before everyone, there will be, Griscom contended, a sharp decline in moral behavior. Even if a family is of good disposition, living in close proximity to many other families with lesser moral standards - an 'impure atmosphere' - will pollute the virtues of the children. Intemperance was another debilitating factor among the poor. One survey showed 111 churches in lower Manhattan and some 6000 pubs to match. Alcoholism was a major health risk among the poor. One of the delights of Griscom's work is his willingness to seek assistance in his studies and in his proposals. For the work on tenement induced diseases, he asked his medical friends to write letters to him about their experiences. For the questions around morality, he asked the Tract Missionaries for their opinions of the effects of poverty on virtue. He was able to provide documentation from reliable sources for his project.

One of the major accomplishments of Griscom's one year in office as City Inspector was his work on death certificates. When he assumed office, the dead could be removed from the city without any documentation of the cause of the disease or violent act that brought on the death. In fact, pre-signed certificates were available so that bodies could be removed without record. Griscom was able to get the law changed - over the veto of the mayor - so that statistical records could be more accurate, providing confirmation of the belief that public health concerns should be central to a government of, by, and for the people.

There was, according to Griscom, a "rout" of the Whig party in New York and he ended his career as City Inspector in 1843. In a letter to Lemuel Shattuck, a Bostonian bookseller and statistician deeply committed to the same public health concerns, Griscom noted that

> My work is unfinished, scarcely begun, and if I must go, the little good I may have done is likely to be lost. But hungry politicians care but little for those things, and I am prepared to walk out.[18]

Griscom maintained a consistent interest in the health of his city. He was appointed Commissioner of Emigration from 1848 to 1851. While serving in this capacity he wrote medical and sanitary rules for the Emigrant Refuge and Hospital on Ward's Island. In 1868 he wrote a report, *Prison Hygiene*, for the New York Prison Association.

The Importance of Air

Griscom focused sharply on the roles that air - good and bad - play in the health of the people. He commented on how much better women looked after a few vacation weeks at the seashore or in the mountains. Friends told him about their children living outside the city who were not sick the past year. His personal experiences with cellar apartments, noted above, were adequate to convince him of the importance of air for health. Also, it must be remembered that physicians of that time 'knew' that bad air - often referred to as malaria or miasma - from rotting garbage, human and animal excreta, slaughter house remnants, and tanneries could produce disease, particularly fevers. Temperature, barometric pressure, and the direction from which the wind blew were other scientific factors to be documented and considered when epidemics were in the offing. So, the qualities of air - putrid both in the cellar and on the street - were epidemiological facts to be detailed.

In an amazing book, *The Uses and Abuses of Air* published in 1850, Griscom addressed again the issues noted above: the importance of good air for development of a healthy people. This book also is a text for the salutary - even salvific - effects of proper ventilation. Griscom was convinced that ventilation in tenements, prisons, refuge centers, and hospitals would prevent much of the disease his office documented. In this book he offered detailed plans for ventilating a wide variety of buildings, especially dwellings. He even patented devices for the proper installation of ventilation both in new dwellings and in existing tenements and public buildings. In his "Concluding Reflections" Griscom pulled together his scientific and his moral reasoning.

As the presence of the atmosphere, in its bountiful abundance and self-maintaining purity, when left to the working of its own natural laws, is universal, so may it be said, that the illustrations of its evil effects, when those laws are interfered with, and its natural freedom restrained, are everywhere to be found, and continually recurring....

God has so plainly written these laws upon all his works, but especially upon that branch of them herein considered, that he who runs may read; nothing but the blindness of ignorance and of obstinate prejudice, can prevent their being seen.[19]

Griscom ends his book with a charge to those responsible for the health of the people.

Let those who have these things in charge, answer to their own consciences how they have discharged their duty, in supplying to the young, the responsibility of whose lives and education they have assumed - A PURE ATMOSPHERE, THE FIRST REQUISITE FOR HEALTHY BODIES AND SOUND MINDS.[20]

Other Interests

In 1859 Griscom became president of the Third National Quarantine Convention. In a report of the Committee on the Internal Hygiene of Cities submitted and written in large part by John Bell, M.D., of Philadelphia, Griscom provided a brief note on the importance of an adequate supply of fresh water and the proper disposal of waste. After writing that "Water should be second only to air in abundance and accessibility," he commented,

> Passing to the subject of sewerage, we have to observe that terrene exhalations in rural localities are a well-known cause of various diseases,...From this cause every city should and can be, made almost wholly free....But however well-paved and sewered a city may be, whereby its natural exhalations are obviated, the formation of *artficial* marshes above the stones of the pavement, and beyond the reach of the sewers, by the accumulation of the offal of men and animals is equally bad, if not worse.[21]

The efforts of Griscom and others were not in vain. In 1866, thanks to a tireless letter-writing campaign by Griscom, the Metropolitan Health Act was passed and New York City had a Board of Health. It was a time of change. Stephen Smith, a New York surgeon and Commissioner of the Metropolitan Board of Health from 1868 to 1875, described those years in his 1911 book, *The City That Was*.

> The Great Awakening, in the middle of the last century, of the people of England, and subsequently, of this country, to the intimate relations of filth, in all forms in and around their dwellings, to the prevalence and fatality of cholera, typhus fever, and other communicable diseases, has restored cleanliness to its ancient imperial position as chief of the virtues, and the most reliable private and public means of conserving health.[22]

In a carefully documented paper presented before the New York Academy of Medicine in 1858 Griscom presented a history of yellow fever epidemics in New York dating from 1618 to a possible one even then, as he spoke. His argument was, again, based upon the causative factor of bad air: summer heat, southwesterly winds, low barometric pressure. He also noted that there was a relationship between the disease and ships arriving in the port carrying sugar from Cuba. In an insightful observation he commented - with some disparagement - on Noah Webster's belief that the absence of yellow fever during the revolutionary war was due to the intervention of Providence in combination with the appearance of comets. Griscom observed that "A more rational solution of the circumstances may, we think, be found in the fact, that during the war nearly all foreign commerce was suspended.[23]"

With later experience, this comment would be verified when, in 1900, a commission under the command of Walter Reed proved the mosquito to be the bearer of the virus responsible for this deadly disease. The virus was not identified until 1928. Since the mosquitoes fly in the air and nest in water, their presumed presence aboard a ship from the Caribbean was quite plausible.

In an exquisitely documented study published in 1868, *Report on Epidemic Cholera and Yellow Fever in the Army of the United States, During the Year 1867,* Brevet Lieut. Col. J. J. Woodward wrote,

> The more thoroughly the facts connected with the spread of yellow fever in the army during 1867 are known, the more strongly they appear to favor the theory of the exotic origin of epidemic yellow fever in the United States....[T]he experience of the medical staff of the army last year furnishes many facts favorable to the doctrine of the portability and transmissibility of the disease, and favorable, therefore, to the establishment of an efficient quarantine in the case of vessels or persons coming from infected places.[24]

Commentary

John H. Griscom is a remarkable model of the life of a person committed to the welfare, not only of the community in which he lived, but of humankind as a whole. He pursued throughout his career as a physician, improvement in the health of the poor and the immigrant. This was unusual for his time, as Charles Rosenberg and Carroll Smith-Rosenberg point out.

> The vast majority of respectable urban Americans - including physicians - found no great difficulty in ignoring the medieval filth and misery which surrounded them....Griscom labored constantly to alert his fellow New Yorkers to the need for sanitary reform. Griscom was for a number of years almost alone among New York physicians in his crusade. This reformist impulse was indeed so atypical in the medical world of the 1840s that it seems logical to explain Griscom's involvement in public health matters not in terms of his role as a physician, but in terms of his being his father's son.[25]

Being his father's son meant that the Quaker influence was a dominant feature in his life. Griscom understood the world to be designed by a benevolent God who provides all that is needed for the comfort and happiness of the created order. The work and the cupidity of humankind produce the catastrophes that are witnessed in the tenements and the work-places of the poor that fill the cities, especially in the days of massive immigration from Europe. Rosenberg and Smith-Rosenberg continued,

> ...Griscom's lasting significance does not rest upon the formal content of his writings. His historical reputation is based on the Quaker physician's tenacious commitment to bettering the living conditions of deprived New Yorkers....Even in his explicitly detailed appeals for public health reorganization, Griscom displayed a persistent tone of moral concern, a guiding dependence upon moral imperatives in shaping his understanding of individual behavior and the place which such reform might play in the upgrading of civic virtue.[26]

Griscom offers us an example of a physician who, working from an established foundation of his interior life, was able to contribute to the welfare of his city and his country without regard for criticism from authorities. His own particular religious and moral underpinnings are not ones that must be followed by others. Rather, our search must be to find a moral and ethical substructure that will provide the courage, the will, and the means to do the work that lies before us in the professions and careers that we choose. Careful study of the intellectual and scientific bases of medicine, knowledge of the social milieu in which medicine is practiced, and commitment to the needs of the communities in which we live and which we serve offer the opportunities to accomplish a realized life. Writing a half-century after Griscom wrote his treatise on the laboring class, Jacob Riis published in 1890 his scathing report on life among the tenements in New York City, *How the Other Half Lives.* This phrase, apparently taken from a 1651 edition of George Herbert's proverbs, *Jacula Prudentum,* "Half the world knows not how the other half lives,"[27] aptly described the city. The profound social gap between the classes seemed insurmountable to Riis, and he called to the people to create a healing bridge between them. He wrote, in the concluding paragraph of his book, about the surging sea of a huge population, mostly immigrant.

> The gap between the classes in which it [the population] surges, unseen, unsuspected by the thoughtless, is widening day by day. No tardy enactment of law, no political expedient, can close it. Against all other dangers our system of government may offer defence and shelter; against

this not. I know of but one bridge that will carry us over safe, a bridge founded upon justice and built of human hearts.[28]

Reform had begun with the work of Griscom and his colleagues, but a final resolution to the perennial health problems associated with poverty, drug dependence, and racial and class prejudices would be delayed into the - as yet not achieved - future.

[1]Jamieson, Duncan R., *Towards a Cleaner New York: John H. Griscom and New York's Public Health, 1830-1870,* Ann Arbor, Michigan, University Microfilms, 1972, i.
[2]Niebuhr, H. Richard, *The Kingdom of God in America,* Harper & Brothers, New York, 1937, 134.
[3]Niebuhr, Ibid., 147.
[4]Griscom, John H., *Memoir of John Griscom, LL.D.,* New York, Robert Carter and Brothers, 1859, 365.
[5]Francis, Samuel W., "Biographical Sketches of Distinguished Living New York Physicians," *Medical & Surgical Reporter,* 15, (1866), 119.
[6]Griscom, John H., *First Lessons in Human Physiology,* New York, Roe Lockwood & Son, 1847, iv.
[7]Richardson, Benjamin Ward, *The Health of Nations, A Review of the Works of Edwin Chadwick,* in two volumes, London, Longmans, Green, and Co., 1887, vol. I, lii.
[8]G,H., "Preface" to Smith, Southwood, *The Philosophy of Health,* 11th edition, London, Longman, Roberts & Green, 1865, v.
[9]Duffy, John, *A History of Public Health in New York City 1625-1866,* New York, Russell Sage Foundation, 1968, 302-3-3.
[10]Griscom, M.D., John H., *The Sanitary Condition Of the Laboring Population of New York,* Harper & Brothers, New York, 1845, 1.
[11]Ibid., 55.
[12]Ibid., 57.
[13]Ibid., 5.
[14]Ibid., 8-9.
[15]Griscom, John H., *Memoir..., op. cit.,* 185.
[16]Dickens, Charles, *American Notes for General Circulation,* London, Chapman and Hall, 1842, vol. I, 191-2.
[17]Ibid., 14.
[18]Cassedy, James H., "The Roots of American Sanitary Reform," *J. Hist. Med.* 30, (1975), 141.
[19]Griscom, John H., *The Uses and Abuses of Air,* New York, J. S. Redfield, Clinton Hall, 1850, 246-247.
[20]Ibid., 249.

[21]Bell, John, M.D., *Report on the Importance and Economy of Sanitary Measures to Cities,* New York, Edmund Jones & Co., 1859, 238-239.
[22]Smith, Stephen, *The City That Was,* New York, Frank Allaben, 1911, 210-211.
[23]Griscom, John H., M.D., "A History, Chronological and Circumstantial, of the Visitations of Yellow Fever At New York," 1858, read before the Academy of Medicine, and printed by permission.
[24]Woodward, J. J., *Report on Epidemic Cholera and Yellow Fever in the Army of the United States, during the Year 1867,* Washington, Government Printing Office, 1868, XVIII.
[25]Rosenberg, Charles E. and Smith-Rosenberg, Carroll, "Pietism and the Origins of the American Public Health Movement: A Note on John H. Griscom and Robert M. Hartley," *J. Hist. Med.& Allied Sc.,* 1968, *23*: 17.
[26]Ibid., 22-23.
[27]Herbert, George, *Jacula prudentem, or Outlandish proverbs, sentences, &c.,* London, Printed by T. M. for T. Garthwait, 1651, No. 907.
[28]Riis, Jacob A., *How the Other Half Lives,* New York, Charles Scribner's Sons, 1890, 296.

Chapter 7

Oliver Wendell Holmes, 1809-1874

Oliver Wendell Holmes was the ultimate Boston Brahmin. This phrase, 'Boston Brahmin,' was actually created by Holmes in his first novel, *Elsie Venner,* published in serial form in the *Atlantic Monthly* magazine beginning in 1859. In the opening chapter he wrote about a New England aristocracy most clearly recognizable in college students. Holmes noted that there were two classes of students: one was "inelegant." "The face is uncouth in feature,...the eye unsympathetic,...the voice is unmusical...." The other class of student is the aristocrat: "his face is smooth, and apt to be pallid, - his features are regular and of a certain delicacy, - his eye is bright and quick,..."[1] Holmes continued by providing the eternal label for this elegant young man who was defined by being a scholar and the son of scholars. "That is exactly what the...young man is. He comes of the *Brahmin caste of New England.*[2]

*S*on of a Calvinist Congregational minister, Abiel Holmes, in Cambridge and a descendent of the Jacksons and Quincys, Holmes was of the caste he described. The years during his childhood were tumultuous ones for the religious sects, particularly in Cambridge where the strains of liberal versus orthodox - Unitarian versus Trinitarian - were powerful. Miriam Rossiter Small, in her 1962 study, *Oliver Wendell Holmes,* wrote,

> The fight was joined with the fierceness of a rearguard action, and Cambridge was a natural battleground, with the dangerous liberal and Unitarian tendencies emanating from college faculty and students. The Reverend Abiel Holmes never turned his back on the orthodox principles in which he had been trained; but, less a theologian than a scholar, he accepted the broadening ways about him in Cambridge naturally and easily;...[3]

The position of his father in the community was ambiguous, leading eventually to his dismissal from his church. Although an orthodox trinitarian in the Puritan tradition, he recognized that the church was living in times of change. But, as Holmes wrote to a friend in 1838, the two great parties which divided our community crowded against him each from his own side - one pressing upon his Calvinist faith, the other upon his liberal principles of intercourse and orderly habits of public ministration, with much care and policy for their own interests, and too little anxiety with regard to him.[4]

The doctrinal squabbles of the day left a permanent mark on Holmes. He remained quizzical about the role of the established church in offering any understanding of the status of the social order. In his novels written later he was critical of the orthodox church, its deacons, and its narrow-minded and self-righteous ministers.

The impact of early exposure to literature is impressive in the story of Holmes. The harsh catechism of Calvinism and the books in his father's study influenced him. John Bunyan's classic, *The Pilgrim's Progress* and a book, apparently sent to his father by a Southern friend called, *The Negro Plot,* established a prejudice in Holmes that it would take years to delete. Well into his thirties he would be taken to task by friends such as James Russell Lowell for his accepting - and ambivalent - positions on slavery and war, poverty, and issues of reform that were becoming crucial national concerns. In an Oration delivered before the New England Society in New York City in 1855, Holmes spoke the following distressing words, first about the American Indian:

The question of interfering races is a very terrible one;...Look at the aboriginal inhabitants of the land we occupy. It pleased the Creator to call into existence this half-filled outline of humanity; this sketch in red crayons of a rudimentary manhood; to keep the continent from being a blank until the true lord of creation should come to claim it. Civilization and Christianity have tried to humanize him, and he proved a dead failure....

And so of the other question between the white and black races....Here, as in the case of the Indians, or any other inferior natural tribe of men, our sympathies will go with our own color first....The white man must be the master in effect, whatever he is in name;...[5]

Holmes seems to have been a rather casual student more noted for quickness than for industry. Eleanor M. Tilton, in her 1947 biography of Holmes, *Amiable Autocrat,* noted that the cigars that Holmes was found to be smoking helped his father to decide to send his errant son to Andover.

Boys did enter Harvard at fifteen, but the minister may have thought his clever, quick-talking son needed the sobering atmosphere of Andover, where a strictly orthodox theological seminary set the tone of the town and the preparatory school. Cambridge was running over with infidels, and...Harvard was more than suspect in its religion.[6]

Holmes did attend Phillips Andover Academy and graduated from Harvard College in 1829, a member of both the Hasty Pudding Club and Phi Beta Kappa. The following year a watershed event occurred. Holmes read, in the September 14 issue of the *Boston Daily Advertiser,* that the Secretary of the Navy was considering dismantling the famous frigate, *Constitution.* Holmes wrote a stirring three-stanza poem, *Old Ironsides,* that achieved national recognition almost instantly, becoming available as broadsides and as handout papers on the streets. The effect was powerful, and resulted in the decision not to destroy the revered memorial. It also confirmed for Holmes his ability as a poet, a commitment that would color the remainder of his long and productive life. His talent and his egocentric desire for public and professional recognition would prove determinative in his dual careers as writer and physician-teacher.

Medical Education

Holmes was undecided what to do for a profession. Certainly the ministry was not a possibility. His biographer, John T. Morse, Jr., noted that

> When Holmes graduated he was still in some doubt as to what should be his calling in life. He went, in a tentative way, into the Dane Law School, and stayed there for a year. But he did not take to his studies with any ardor, and scanty trace of any influence of this twelvemonth is to be noted in his writings....In fact, however, he had not started on the right road; he soon found it out, and stopped at the first milestone.[7]

Holmes began the study of medicine in the winter of 1830-31 at Harvard Medical School where the faculty numbered six at that time (Winslow Lewis, Demonstrator of Anatomy had just been added). There was no teaching in physiology, and the microscope was not in evidence. Five courses of lectures were offered in two series from November through January: Theory and Practice of Medicine, Anatomy and Surgery, Obstetrics and Medical Jurisprudence, Chemistry, and Materia Medica. A college education was not a requirement; students were expected to have a knowledge of Latin and elementary physics. Holmes also attended the private school on

Tremont Street that had the same faculty as Harvard. These private schools, for those who could afford to attend them, filled in some of the gaps so apparent in the limited curricula of university and proprietary schools. James Jackson, Sr., a physician whom Holmes would revere throughout his life, was the senior member of the faculty. Holmes probably received as good an education in medicine as was available in the United States at that time. His true career destination was writing, but he would not fulfill that goal until later in his life. Holmes, in commenting on his choice of medicine, writes, "What determined me to give up Law and apply myself to Medicine I can hardly say, but I had from the first looked upon that year's study as an experiment. At any rate, I made the change, and soon found myself introduced to new scenes and new companionships.[8]"

These "new scenes and new companionships" would have as their center the figure of James Jackson, Sr., M.D. who would be an example of the ultimate physician for Holmes. In an Introductory Lecture delivered before the Harvard medical class in 1867, Holmes began by pointing out the essential role of bedside teaching versus lecture for students of medicine. He continued with a discussion of the teaching methods of former physicians at the medical school and the chief elements of their instruction that were important. All this led up to his eulogy for James Jackson, attributing to him the highest praise. A physician who was devoted to his patients, who stayed with them as they struggled with their diseases, Jackson was acutely aware of the need for kindness as well as skill. Holmes wrote that Jackson

> used to insist on one small point with a certain philological precision, namely, the true meaning of the word "cure." He would have it that to *cure* a patient was simply to *care* for him....such devotion as this is only to be looked for in the man who gives himself wholly up to the business of healing, who considers Medicine itself a Science, or if not a science, is willing to follow it as an art,...[9]

Holmes went to Paris in 1834, along with a number of other Americans who would subsequently, as a result of their education, transform their understanding of medicine and of themselves as physicians. William Osler wrote,

> In the thirties a very remarkable body of young Americans studied in Paris, chiefly under the great Louis - Oliver Wendell Holmes, James Jackson, Jr., Henry I. Bowditch, and George C. Shattuck, from Boston,...They brought back to this country scientific methods of work and habits of accurate, systematic observation, and they had caught also, what was much more valuable, some of his inspiring enthusiasm.[10]

For Holmes, Pierre Louis was the leading teacher of the Paris School. His dedication to accurate diagnosis confirmed at autopsy, his perseverance in both study and patient care, and his acceptance of the requirement to teach were major factors in Holmes' committed loyalty to Louis.   Like Holmes, Louis had attended law school for a year before deciding to become a physician.   One wonders whether the two men discussed their choices of career.

In a letter to his parents from Paris Holmes commented on his dedicated time to study. His words do not sound like ones he might have written in law school.

I am, as usual, all medicine, getting up at seven and going to hospitals, cutting up, hearing lectures, soaking, infiltrating in the springs of knowledge.   There is a great deal more to be done than I was inclined to suppose, but the more the better, when one gets into good working trim.[11]

The opportunities for learning were remarkable when one recalls the apprenticeship model current in the United States at that time. Holmes was explicit:

...I have undisputed entrance at all times to two wards, containing together a hundred beds, generally full, where I examine and pound and overhaul the patients before even Louis or his *interne* have seen them.[12]

In a letter to John O. Sargent, Holmes noted the personal impact of this work, again quite different from his law school experiences.

The nature of the studies which I am pursuing, the singular advantages which I am at present enjoying, and the number of objects which absolutely require my attention have induced - have forced me rather, to forbid myself any diversion from the path of my professional studies.[13]

One of the more remarkable aspects of the education available to all students was the ability to purchase the bodies of the recently deceased at the cemetery of Clamart for dissection and for practicing operations. At noon each day the students paid fifty sous for a subject and, as Holmes writes, "before evening we had cut him into inch pieces." He continued,

Now all this can hardly be done anywhere in the world but at Paris, - in England and America we can *dissect*, but rarely operate upon the subject, while here one who knows how to use his hands, and who gives his attention exclusively to the subject for a time,..becomes an expert operator in a few weeks.[14]

The Professor

Holmes returned to Boston in the late winter of 1835 and received his M.D. degree from Harvard in 1836. A requirement for his degree was a dissertation, and he wrote one on acute pericarditis which he submitted January 12, 1836. This paper is essentially a summary of the writings of others on this disease. It does conclude with an important observation on the role of bloodletting. After noting 'copious depletion' used by M. Bouillaud, Holmes quoted a "Dr. Fordyce from his Dissertation on Fever, p. 184," who had rarely lost a patient in the past fifteen years of his practice. Fordyce wrote,

> In this period, he has entirely left off bleeding in acure rheumatism; and has not lost above two or three patients, although he has treated several hundreds in this disease.[15]

Holmes was careful, in his final summation, to note that no other authors had had this experience. He declined to draw any conclusion himself.

Holmes joined the Massachusetts Medical Society and began what was to be a desultory medical practice. He was appointed physician to the Boston Dispensary, a charity hospital. In 1838 he was appointed professor of anatomy at Dartmouth College, a position he held for several years, returning finally to Harvard in 1847 as Parkman Professor of Anatomy and Physiology. In his Introductory Lecture to the entering medical class on November 3, 1847, Holmes commented that one who is appointed professor

> is bound, by the most solemn obligations, to the young men who trust some of their dearest interests in his hands, to the University which lends him the authority of her venerable name, to the community by whom that institution is protected and cherished, and, above all, to the great Taskmaster who has granted him an honorable and grateful sphere of labor.[16]

Holmes continued in his lecture with a delightful series of comments on the difficulties of making certain medical topics easily presentable as lectures. There are days, he said, when

> The memory sometimes neglects its duty, the imagination droops, the tongue will not perform its office, and as from an untuned instrument, a few discordant notes are all that can be obtained instead of the expected harmony.[17]

He concluded with a promise to work hard to help the students learn, the University prosper, and provide a good legacy for those who would follow him in his work. Holmes was to remain professor of anatomy until his retirement in 1882. He was a remarkable lecturer - witty, sharp, and inventive. He was assigned the last lecture slot of the day when most students were either asleep or had left for the day. Holmes was able to hold them captive with his style.

Early Medical Writings

In 1836 Holmes received the Boylston Medical Prize awarded for writing an essay on an assigned topic. He shared the 1836 prize with two other authors writing on the value of the findings of external examination of the patient by auscultation, percussion, and succussion (shaking). Holmes commented on the difficulties some older physicians had in using these techniques, preferring to rely on palpation, the condition of the tongue, and taking the pulse. He recognized the wariness many felt toward the introduction of novelties.

It was perfectly natural that they should look with suspicion upon this introduction of medical machinery [the stethescope] among the old hard working operatives; that they should for a while smile at its pretensions; and when its use began to creep in among them, that they should observe and signalize all the errors and defects which happened in its practical application.[18]

Holmes won two Boylston prizes in 1837, one for a paper on neuralgia that was a review of contemporary literature and experience, the other an extended history and review of malaria in New England. For the latter he had carefully collected data from many physicians throughout the region. The essay was highly praised after its publication in 1838.

The growing medical profession of Homoeopathy was a target for Holmes' sharp tongue. In February 1842 he delivered two lectures before the Boston Society for the Diffusion of Useful Knowledge titled, "Homoeopathy and Its Kindred Delusions." His hope was to inform the public about one of the major quackeries of the day. This talk, after publication, received a mixed review from the newspapers and the press. Discontent with current medical practice had made the gentleness of homoeopathic medicine attractive to a large number of persons distressed by bloodletting, purging, and leeches. In his concluding remarks, after pointing out the apparent inconsistencies, confusions, and absurdities of Hahnemann's theories, he said,

> Such is the pretended science of Homoeopathy, to which you are asked to trust your lives and the lives of those dearest to you. A mingled mass of perverse ingenuity, of tinsel erudition, of imbecile credulity, and of artful misrepresentation, too often mingled in practice, if we may trust the authority of its founder, with heartless and shameless imposition....If it should claim a longer existence, it can only be by falling into the hands of the sordid wretches who wring their bread from the cold grasp of disease and death in the hovels of ignorant poverty.[19]

William Osler, in his essay on Holmes, wrote that the "essay on Homeopathy remains one of the most complete exposures of that therapeutic fad. There is no healthier or more stimulating writer to students and to young medical men.[20] Holmes used his Paris experiences to disprove any theory of disease or of treatment that did not have what he considered a 'scientific' basis. The concept that miniscule amounts of drugs could have any effect was not a consideration. He was also significantly influenced by the work of his friend and contemporary, Jacob Bigelow, who, in 1835, published a landmark paper on self-limited diseases, strongly opposing 'heroic therapies.' Holmes also wrote a poem, "Compliments to Homoeopathists," that spoke to the folly of their profession. This poem, and a talented reply, "A Return Compliment to Allopathists,' by [C.D.] were printed in The American Homoeopathic Review for June-July 1866. The cap-stone of Holmes' career in medicine, however, was his 1843 paper on puerperal fever, also known popularly as child-bed fever.

Puerperal Fever

In June of 1842, at a meeting of the Boston Society for Medical Improvement, an obstetrician reported on thirteen cases of puerperal fever. In the fall of the year more cases were presented, and, by December Holmes was reading avidly the medical journals. For some fifty years, the contagiousness of this killer of women just delivered - and their babies - had been hinted at. Doctors and medical students who performed their autopsies occasionally died. Holmes' readings and collection of cases from other physicians confirmed his belief in the contagious nature of the disease. In February of 1843 Holmes presented his findings in a talk before the Boston Society for Medical

Improvement. This was published in a short-lived journal, but did receive positive responses in the profession. In the beginning of his paper Holmes makes the italicized statement, *"The disease known as puerperal fever is so far contagious as to be frequently carried from patient to patient by physicians and nurses.*[21] Holmes went on to quote a Doctor Gordon of Aberdeen who, in a treatise published in 1795, clearly proved the contagiousness of the disease and its transmission by practitioners. Gordon's conclusion was that "these facts fully prove that the cause...was a specific contagion, or infection altogether unconnected with a noxious constitution of the atmosphere."[22] Holmes concluded his passionate and stirring essay with a list of precautions and warnings for practitioners to help save the lives of women, many of whom were terrified of pregnancy because of the threat of death. This paper stirred a controversy among obstetricians who were shocked that any other doctor could implicate them in the deaths of their patients. The paper was printed a number of times, but it was not until the early years of the 1850s when two renowned Philadelphia obstetricians, Hodge and Meigs, wrote articles condemning the idea of contagion, that Holmes re-published the paper. It was then that the full positive impact of Holmes' work was noted and praised, and its significance acclaimed as one of the most memorable medical reports in our history. The evidence was in, and Holmes stuck to his theory. In an 1894 talk before the Johns Hopkins Medical Society William Osler said,

> The results of his studies are summed up in a series of eight conclusions, and the strong ground which he took may be gathered from this sentence in the last one: 'The time has come when the existence of a private pestilence in the sphere of a single physician should be looked upon not as a misfortune but a crime.'[23]

Other Writings

Holmes was a occasional speaker at Harvard medical commencements. He obviously enjoyed this opportunity to display his skills in writing and his performance capabilities 'on stage.' But he was also a careful thinker about the moral, as well as the professional, aspects of medical practice. In his 1858 address to the graduates he pointed out to them that once a doctor, always a doctor. "You can unfrock a clergyman and unwed a husband, but you can never put off the title you have just won." He went on to offer two counsels.

Form a distinct PLAN for life, including duties to fulfil, virtues to practice, powers to develop, knowledge to attain, graces to acquire....nothing else goes on well without a plan;...
DUTY draws the great circle which includes all else within it....If performed in the right spirit, there is no higher worship than the unpurchased service of the medical priesthood.

Holmes continued with a discussion of the virtue of truth-telling. Doctors are, as he said, "expected to know the truth, and to be ready to tell it." Part of the responsibility of knowing and revealing the truth is the demand that the physician be true, first to the patient, and then to himself. Finally, Holmes spoke to his belief that

Charity is the eminent virtue of the medical profession...a virtue which I am content to leave you to learn from those who have gone before you, and whose footprints you will find in the path of every haunt of stricken humanity.[24]

Holmes repeatedly stressed, not only the relationships between student and teacher, but also the similarity among all. In his Introductory Lecture before the medical class at Harvard on November 6, 1861, he pointed out that

This day belongs...not to myself and my recollections, but to all of us who teach and all of you who listen, whether experts in our specialties or aliens to their mysteries,...
SCIENCE is the topography of ignorance. From a few elevated points we triangulate vast spaces, enclosing infinite unknown details....
The best part of our knowledge is that which teaches us where knowledge leaves off and ignorance begins....
That which is true of every subject is especially true of that branch of knowledge which deals with living beings.[25]

Holmes concluded his lecture with his advice that disputations among physicians lead to little. There are always those who oppose any new understanding or interpretation. One must be sure that the work is correct and will be able to stand to its own defense. Opposition is important in clarifying belief.

Later Writing

At the end of his professional career in 1882 Holmes gave a farewell address to the medical school at Harvard. Titled, "Some of my Early Teachers," it is revealing - and not unexpected - that Pierre Louis played the major role in forming Holmes' medical education. Noting the "addiction" that the students had to Louis, Holmes wrote of the "reverence, I might almost say idolatry," they felt.

> If I summed up the lessons of Louis in two expressions, they would be these;...Always make sure that you form a distinct and clear idea of the matter you are considering. Always avoid vague approximations where exact estimates are possible;...
> [W]hat Louis did was this: he showed by a strict analysis of numerous cases that bleeding did not strangle, - *jugulate* was the word then used, - acute diseases, especially pneumonia. This was not a reform, - it was a revolution....[26]

Holmes noted that one of the major learning experiences at the side of Louis was that many diseases are self-limited, and that patients often get well by themselves. This was, in 1835, explicitly developed in the writings of Jacob Bigelow, a leading reformer of the practice of medicine in his day. Holmes became convinced that drugging is often useless, if not expressly harmful. Of importance also to students of medicine in any era is Holmes's observation in his Farewell Address that the fascination the students felt toward the 'science' of Louis often kept them from attending to other teachers - Broussais, Andral, and others - who taught therapy, caring for patients. Holmes was concerned that the negative facts about bloodletting and leeches displaced the positive facts of a caring practice, that

> There is one part of their business which certain medical practitioners are apt to forget;, namely, that what they should most of all try to do is to ward off disease, to alleviate suffering, to preserve life, or at least to prolong it if possible.[27]

The fascination of students for scientific advances over bedside attendance remains to this day. Even though Louis also used common heroic therapies, he did so less often and in a steadily diminishing way, finally convinced of the uselessness, even harm, of the procedure.

Other Interests

In an address before the Annual Meeting of the Massachusetts Medical Society in 1860 Holmes made what is perhaps his most often quoted statement from his medical writings; "[I]f the whole materia medica, *as now used,* could be sunk to the bottom of the sea, it would be all the better for mankind - and all the worse for the fishes.[28]"

He had, earlier in the Address, noted that

> There is no offence, then, or danger in expressing the opinion, that, after all which has been said, the community is still over-dosed. The best proof of it is, that no families take so little medicine as those of doctors, except those of apothecaries, and that old practitioners are more sparing of active medicines than younger ones.[29]

Holmes pressed for care in evaluating the effects of therapies, pointing out that we are apt to remember only the successes and to base our advice on them, selectively forgetting our failures. Hygiene was placed high on the list of functions of the doctor as discerner of ways to prevent diseases.

Of course, to the general reader, Holmes is best known for his series of articles that appeared in the *Atlantic Monthly* over a period of years, the Breakfast Table series. In these revealing essays, the Autocrat, the Professor, the Poet, and one who converses Over the Teacups discussed most of the issues of the day, public and personal, that readers waited eagerly to see appear each month. It was the conveyed sense that the reader was actually talking with the author that led to its popularity. Although he had written two pieces for the *New England Magazine* in 1831 and in 1832 called, *Autocrat of the Breakfast-Table*, they cannot be compared with the pieces written twenty-five years later. In the first number, published in November 1857, Holmes described the nature of conversation so important to the author.

> This business of conversation is a very serious matter....There are men of *esprit* who are excessively exhausting to some people. They are the talkers who have what may be called *jerky* minds. Their thoughts do not run in the natural order of sequence....After a jolting half-hour with one of these jerky companions, talking with a dull friend affords great relief. It is like taking the cat in your lap after holding a squirrel.[30]

Holmes also wrote three novels - again in monthly installments - that received very mixed reviews. An underlying theme in the writings of Holmes is his disavowal of the faith of his father. Small noted in her biography of Holmes that he

> struck against the dark creed of the Calvinists, which he discarded in favor of a God of love, a God that granted human beings Thought, Conscience, and Will to use for their own growth and happiness as much as for God's glory.[31]

Holmes seemed to have grasped the importance of the new sciences and the new philosophies for the coming generations. There was more to caring for patients than prescribing doses of medicine. Even though he did not practice medicine for most of his professional life, he was a careful observer of the contemporary scene, and he wrote about - and to - the necessity of the physician to be alert to change and to self-definition provided by searching insight into the self.

The life and the works of Oliver Wendell Holmes offer the reader a cautionary tale. In his aging he was aware that he was now on the sidelines of science and political theory and practice. A friend of Lowell, Emerson, Whittier, Longfellow, and William James, he was also exposed to the thoughts and the practices of the leading physicians and surgeons of his day. Holmes studied the works of Darwin, incorporating them into his understanding of his world. He had questions, in his old age, about his interests being in disparate fields; perhaps he would have been more effective if he had limited himself to medicine *or* poetry *or* the novel. He did proceed on two levels of significant engagement with his culture: he tried to bring scientific knowledge to the public in an understandable way, and he attempted to remain aware of advances in the medical sciences so that he would be contemporary with his students and colleagues. The work of William James on the interplay between psychology and religion was innovative in that day and it interested Holmes. He praised the work on which James had embarked, seeing in it new ways in which the human venture could be interpreted.

Commentary

Oliver Wendell Holmes offers us a biographical study that can awaken us to our own lives. Highly intelligent and interested in his world, he was also exquisitely self-centered and self-directed. As a conversationalist he could not be silenced; he sought praise and confirmation from all sources; he was delighted to be flattered, seeking it from colleagues, from the public, and from the press; he wrote numerous poems to celebrate various events, medical and public, and he cultivated the praise of his students. He also struggled in his youth against a repressive theology and was able to free himself to become a liberated person. He knew the value of education, seeking out the best of his day in the Paris School, allying himself with its outstanding teacher, Pierre Louis. Holmes was loyal to his family, to his friends, and to his medical school where he taught for many decades. He can well be considered a reliable teacher for us.

William Osler wrote, in his essay on Holmes, that

> There is no healthier or more stimulating writer to students and to young medical men. With an entire absence of nonsense, with rare humor and unfailing kindness, and with that delicacy of feeling characteristic of a member of the Brahmin class, he has permanently enriched the literature of the race.[32]

[1]Holmes, Oliver Wendell, *Elsie Venner,* Houghton, Mifflin and Company, Boston, 1861, 3.

[2]Ibid., 4.

[3]Small, Miriam Rossiter, *Oliver Wendell Holmes,* Twayne Publishers, Inc., New York, 1962, 30.

[4]Holmes, Oliver Wendell, February 21, 1838 letter to the Reverend William Jenks, quoted in Tilton, Eleanor M., *Amiable Autocrat,* New York, Henry Schuman, 1947, 148.

[5]Holmes, Oliver Wendell, *Oration Delivered Before the New England Society, December 22, 1855,* publisher unknown, 41-43.

[6]Tilton, Eleanor Marguerite, *Amiable Autocrat: a Biography of Dr. Oliver Weldell Holmes,* Henry Schuman, New York, 1947, 25.

[7]Morse, Jr., John Torrey, *Life and Letters of Oliver Wendell Holmes,* vol. I, Houghton, Milflin and Company, Boston, 78-79.

[8]Holmes, Oliver Wendell, "Some of My Early Teachers," *Medical Essays 1842-1882,* Houghton, Mifflin and Company, Boston, 1888, 424.

[9]Holmes, Oliver Wendell, "Scholastic and Bedside Teaching," *Medical Essays,* Ibid., 307-308.

[10]Osler, William, "Oliver Wendell Holmes," *An Alabama Student and Other Biographical Essays,* London, Oxford University Press, 1908, 58.

[11]Morse, *op. cit.,* 120-121.

[12]Ibid., 143.

[13]Ibid., 146.

[14]Ibid., 151-152.

[15]Holmes, Oliver Wendell, *A Dissertation on Acute Pericarditis,* Boston, The Welch Bibliophilic Society, 1937, 39.

[16]Holmes, Oliver Wendell, *An Introductory Lecture, Delivered at the Massachusetts Medical College, November 3, 1847,* Boston, William D. Ticknor & Company, 1847, 26-27.

[17]Ibid., 31.

[18]Holmes, Oliver Wendell, "Dissertation by Oliver W. Holmes," *Library of Practical Medicine,* volume VII, Boston, Perkins & Marvin, 1836, 195.

[19]Holmes, Oliver Wendell, "Homoeopathy and Its Kindred Delusions," *Medical Essays 1842-1882, op. cit., 101.*

[20]Osler, "Oliver Wendell Holmes," *op. cit.,* 66.

[21]Holmes, Oliver Wendell, "The Contagiousness of Puerperal Fever," *Medical Essays 1842-1882, op. cit.,* 131.

[22]Ibid., 135.

[23]Osler, "Oliver Wendell Holmes," *op. cit.,* 62.

[24]Holmes, Olver Weldell, *Valedictory Address to the Medical Graduates of Harvard University,* March 10, 1858, Boston, David Clapp, 1858, 3, 4, 9.

[25]Holmes, Oliver Wendell, *Border Lines of Knowledge in Some Provinces of Medical Science,* Boston, Ticknor and Fields, 1862, 6-7.

[26]Holmes, *Medical Essays, 1842-1882, op. cit.,* 431-433.

[27]Ibid., 433-434.

[28]Tilton, *op. cit.,* 255.

[29]Holmes, Oliver Wendell, *An Address Delivered Before the Massachusetts Medical Society, May 30, 1860,* Boston, Ticknor and Fields, 1860, 17-18.

[30]Holmes, Oliver Wendell, *The Autocrat of the Breakfast-Table, The "Breakfast-Table" Series,* London, George Routledge and Sons, 1889, 7.

[31]Small, *op. cit.,* 60.

[32]Osler, *op. cit.,* 66-67.

Chapter 8

Elizabeth Blackwell, 1821-1910

Elizabeth Blackwell was the first woman to receive the degree of Doctor of Medicine in the United States. She graduated first in her class, with 129 men, from Geneva Medical College in Western New York State in 1849 after completing the required two Fall terms of study. She had a remarkable career in an era of confusion and confrontation over issues of self-definition and professional identification in both American and European medicine. Conservative forces vigorously resisted allowing women to enter the profession. The evolving fields of laboratory physiology and bacteriology, and the explosive impact of Darwinism threatened the self-understanding of the 'art of the doctor,' calling into question the very foundations of medical education, training, and practice. Blackwell's personal life and professional career present critiques of the established and accepted understanding of the practice of medicine in the second half of nineteenth century United States. Her career stands, in part, in a polar relation to that of another woman physician whose career I will present, Mary Putnam Jacobi. Some twenty years younger, she was a colleague of Blackwell who understood the roles of women in the family, in society, and in medical education and practice quite differently.

The Early Years

Elizabeth Blackwell was born in Bristol, England, one of eight children. Her father owned a sugar refinery, was a Dissenter from the Church of England, and an Abolitionist. An interesting comment on human capacity for self-deception is found in a footnote to a 1947 paper by Laurence G. Roth on Elizabeth Blackwell.

> As an aside to the student of human nature, the following is of interest: The Blackwell family had voluntarily given up the use of sugar because it was a slave product. However, the fact that they considered sugar a slave product did not prevent them from gaining their livelihood by refining sugar.[1]

Samuel Blackwell was convinced that boys and girls should be well educated, attending all classes together. Therefore his children were taught at home, receiving a broad and excellent education that included the classics and contemporary foreign languages, and stressed the centrality of the moral life. In her later years Elizabeth was recognized as a very well educated person. Economic and political crises in England persuaded Samuel Blackwell to move to America in 1832. They settled in New York City, moving to Cincinnati in 1838 when Elizabeth was seventeen. Her father died shortly thereafter at the age of forty-eight, leaving the family with little money. The children scattered to jobs in teaching and business to support the family. Elizabeth became a teacher.

Cincinnati was a stronghold of the Abolitionist Movement, the hometown of the Lyman Beecher family and Harriet Beecher Stowe. William H. Channing, one of the founders of a communal living arrangement - Brook Farm - in Concord, Massachusetts, was the local minister. These friends provided a milieu for Elizabeth that encouraged social action, personal independence, and the importance of intellectual growth without regard to gender. Elizabeth's personal story is complex. Her powerful religious beliefs supported her commitments to social and political reform. The combination of her puritanical faith with its stern understanding of a moral social order and its wariness of human desires and passions, her excellent education, her expressed hope to do good work in a troubled world, and her apparently suppressed sexuality led her to consider medicine as a career. There were, at that time, no women allopathic physicians. Her decision to become a doctor was the result of several powerful experiences.

The Path to an M. D.

In 1844, at the age of 23, Blackwell was teaching in a small school in Henderson, Kentucky. Distressed by the presence of slavery and the tedium of teaching, she returned to Cincinnati. She enjoyed the social and intellectual life, and was also aware of her attraction to young men, an emotion that distressed her. In her 1895 autobiography, *Pioneer Work for Women,* Blackwell presented the events that led to her decision to apply to medical school.

It was at this time [1845 in Cincinnati] that the suggestion of studying medicine was first presented to me by a lady friend. This friend finally died of a painful disease, the delicate nature of which made the methods of treatment a constant suffering to her. She once said to me: "You are fond of study, have health and leisure; why not study medicine? If I could have been treated by a lady doctor, my worst sufferings would have been spared me." But I at once repudiated the suggestion as an impossible one, saying that I hated everything connected with the body, and could not bear the sight of a medical book....

So I resolutely tried for weeks to put the idea suggested by my friend away; but it constantly recurred to me. Other circumstances forced upon me the necessity of devoting myself to some absorbing occupation. I became impatient of the disturbing influence exercised by the other sex. I had always been extremely susceptible to this influence....[W]henever I became sufficiently intimate with any individual to be able to realize what a life association might mean, I shrank from the prospect, disappointed or repelled.

I find in my journal of that time the following sentence, written during an acute attack:-

I felt more determined than ever to become a physician, and thus place a strong barrier between me and all ordinary marriage. I must have something to engross my thoughts, some object in life which will fill this vacuum and prevent this sad wearing away of the heart.[2]

Her efforts during the next two years took on the character of what she would call a moral struggle. There was the need for a commitment so that she could bypass marriage. Her education and family environment provided the will power to succeed in what seemed a futile enterprise to her female friends and almost all male physicians: to overcome the strong resistance of medical schools to admit women as students. To earn money for her anticipated enrollment in medical school she went to Asheville, North Carolina to teach music in a small school. She arrived at the end of June 1845. Her brothers who drove her there by carriage left and she was alone in her room.

Doubt and dread of what might be before me gathered in my mind. I was overwhelmed with sudden terror of what I was undertaking. In an agony of mental despair I cried out, "Oh God, help me, support me! Lord Jesus, guide, enlighten me!"...Suddenly, overwhelmingly, an answer came,...a spiritual influence so joyful, gentle, but powerful surrounded me that the despair which had overwhelmed me vanished. All doubt as to the future, all hesitation as to the rightfulness of my purpose, left me and never in after-life returned. I *knew* that, however insignificant my individual effort might be, it was in a right direction,...this unusual experience at the outset of my medical career, has had a lasting and marked effect on my whole life....[3]

In the summer of 1847 Blackwell sailed to Philadelphia, considered the center of medical education in the United States. There she took private anatomy lessons from a Dr. Allen, and began her interviews with physicians associated with the four schools in that city. At the time there were forty-two all-male medical schools in the United States to which she could apply. Applications to all the standard schools on the Eastern seaboard were rejected. While waiting to hear she attended lectures and observed patients with a Quaker physician on the faculty at Jefferson, a Dr. Warrington who kindly supported Blackwell's efforts. She then "obtained a complete list of all the smaller schools of the Northern States, 'country schools,' as they were called."[4] She applied to twelve and was accepted at Geneva Medical College near Syracuse. [This school would become the medical school of Syracuse University.] She began her studies there in November 1847.

Dr. Stephen Smith, a New York surgeon and a Commissioner of Health for the City of New York in the 1860s and 1870s, was a student at Geneva when Blackwell arrived. In his opening address at a convocation in memory of the Blackwell sisters in 1911 arranged by The Women's Medical Association of New York City, Smith commented on the school.

> Being located in the country, the class of students was largely made up of the sons of farmers, tradesmen, and mechanics. A common saying among the people of that vicinity was, that a boy who proved unfit for anything else must become a Doctor....
> Under these circumstances the class contained a large element of rude and uncouth country youths, whose love of "fun" far exceed their love of learning.[5]

Smith continued and described how the faculty, completely opposed to admitting a woman but not wanting to officially vote that way, left the vote up to the students who, surprisingly, voted to accept Blackwell as a student. She lived and studied isolated from others, but accomplished her goals completely. In fact, her presence often forced instructors to modify the coarse language often permissible when discussing human anatomical parts. Her teachers seemed to have been pleased with her presence.

During her spring term in 1850 Blackwell worked at Blockley Almshouse (later Blockley Hospital [Old Blockley] of the University of Pennsylvania Medical School.) This was an important experience for her. Ishbel Ross, in her 1949 biography of Blackwell, *Child of Destiny,* wrote,

She was assigned to the women's syphilitic department, and this was the starting point of her life-long fight on venereal disease and the white-slave traffic. Many of the inmates were the dregs of the slums. Others were innocent immigrant servants, who had been seduced by their employers. When one threw herself from a window, Elizabeth wrote in her diary: "All this is horrible! Women must really open their eyes to it. I am convinced that *they* must regulate the matter. But how?[6]

Blackwell graduated at the head of her class of 130 students in January 1849, the first woman in the United States to receive an M.D. Her commencement was noted by 'Punch' in London with a poem, the final stanza of which said,

> For Doctrix Blackwell - that's the way
>   To dub in rightful gender -
> In her profession, ever may
>   Prosperity attend her!
> 'Punch' a gold-handled parasol
>   Suggests for presentation
> To one so well deserving all
>   Esteem and admiration.[7]

The Training Continues

Blackwell realized that her medical education was far from complete so she returned to Philadelphia where, as she wrote, "I was politely received by the heads of the profession...as a professional sister." On March 6, 1849 she wrote in her journal,

> A morning of great gratification; welcomed cordially to the university, and afterwards heard Doctors Jackson, Hodges, Gibson, Chapman, and Horner lecture. Drs. Lee and Ford were with me, the former quite in spirits at my reception.[8]

Although she visited the university hospital, she was excluded from any practical medical experiences. She had been advised, even before going to Geneva, to go to Paris, the city on the forefront of clinical investigation, for her medical education. In the spring of 1849 she sailed for France, stopping for a visit in England. She was escorted on tours of several hospitals and museums, arriving in Paris in May. A Boston physician had given her a sealed letter of introduction to Pierre Louis. Louis came to visit her, listened to her desire to study, and then advised that she attend La Maternité. He seemed cool and distant; this was soon explained when he returned the letter of introduction to Blackwell. Written in very poor French, it was interpreted by Louis as an insult. Blackwell attended some public medical lectures, met Claude Bernard, but it was very apparent that her M.D. degree was not accepted, and that she would not be admitted to study medicine and surgery. Giving in to the obvious, she did apply to La Maternité' where she worked for a year, essentially as a young woman learning to be a midwife. She wrote,

> On June 30 [1849] I entered La Maternité: my residence there was an invaluable one at that stage of the medical campaign, when no hospitals, dispensaries, or practical *cliniques* were open to women....The system of instruction, both theoretical and practical, was a remarkable illustration of that genius for organisation which belongs to the French. Every moment of time was appropriated; no distraction of books, newspapers, or other than medical works were allowed; lectures, wardwork, drills, and *cliniques* were arranged from morning to night with no confusion, but no pause; and the comprehension and progress of each pupil was constantly tested by examination.[9]

Her education there in obstetrics was excellent, as one would expect from her description. Unfortunately, during her stay she developed a severe eye infection, probably ophthalmia neonatorum - a gonococcal infection - that she got when, syringing the eyes of an infected infant, pus splashed on her face. She had an emotionally jarring response to this infection, eventually losing her vision in that eye, and it was surgically removed.

Blackwell left Paris and was accepted as a student at St. Bartholomew's Hospital in London by James Paget (1814-1899). This outstanding surgeon and pathologist was considered a co-founder of the then new specialty of pathology; he was knighted in 1871. It was he who pointed out to Blackwell that she would encounter far more prejudice from women than from men, a fact that was unfortunately confirmed in her work in England. She was told by other women that they would *never* accept a woman as their physician. She was, however, well accepted by the staff, made a number of friends in London, and felt comfortable in her new role. She considered herself ready to return to the United States and begin the practice of medicine. William H. Welch, former Dean of the Johns Hopkins School of Medicine, spoke at the meeting held in memory of the Blackwell sisters in 1911. He commented on the influence of Blackwell becoming a physician:

[T]his entrance to the profession of medicine marked the opening of a larger sphere of interest and of work to women in general. It is somewhat curious that the entrance upon the practice of medicine should have been the first event in what is spoken of as the "woman's movement," for the movement for the higher education of women, and various other movements of a kindred character were subsequent to this.[10]

To justify placing Blackwell as an important - even defining - figure in American medical history I will discuss two parts of her professional life that not only determined who she was as a person, but point up the revolutionary changes that occurred in the latter half of the nineteenth century: 1), the woman doctor, and, 2), the hygienist.

The Woman Doctor

Before recounting the professional journey of Elizabeth Blackwell, a look at the rise of feminism in mid-nineteenth century America will set the stage. There were divergent views, even among women, as to the roles women could, and should, play. For some, domestic reform was the key issue: making home life more compatible with the good life in matters economic, sexual, and child-rearing. This view was supported by the belief that women were more sympathetic and compassionate, and much less driven by carnal desires than men. A common belief ascribed to by many was that women were not sexually passionate, and that female orgasm was a rarity. It was recommended by some activists that women be given complete control over the frequency of intercourse. Underlying this recommendation were several realities: 1), inadequate and ineffective birth control measures; 2), the very present threat of death from childbed fever due to dirty hands of doctors and midwives; and 3), the sharp divide between the household duties of the woman and the work and civic duties of the man so clearly prescribed by the culture. Regina Markell Morantz-Sanchez, in her Introduction to her 1985 book, *Sympathy and Science,* wrote that some feminists

believed that women's work would best be confined to those concerns which were obviously "feminine" - the education of the young, the safe-keeping of social morality, moral and religious uplift among the poor, municipal housekeeping, bringing the benefits of medical science to bear on family life. Most feminists, especially in the nineteenth century, believed that women should enter public life because they had a unique contribution to make that men could not.[11]

The differences between the sexes was never stressed more than in the feminine capacity for sympathy. One of the strongest arguments posed by women for their acceptance into the medical profession was the compassion they would bring to it. The central argument was that the feminine role in the family translated well into the public sphere, regardless of the work that was done. Women physicians played an important part in determining the course of feminism. Virginia G. Drachman, in her 1976 doctoral thesis, *Women Doctors and the Women's Medical Movement: Feminism and Medicine, 1850-1895,* wrote that

> In contrast to male doctors who defined ill health as inherent to womanhood, women doctors argued that it was the social conditions of women's lives that destroyed their health....[T]hey knew from their patients that the over-work of working class women, the ennui of middle class women and inability of all women to control their reproductive capacities were all part of the explanation for the deterioration in women's health.[12]

Women physicians, learning through their accepted intimacy with their women patients about their private lives, were able to add strong foundational arguments to the reforming drive for equality and opportunity for women in America.

Achieving her M.D. degree was the first of many hurdles placed in the career path of Blackwell. Her rejection in Philadelphia and her assigned position as an aide in La Maternité were foretastes of her reception in New York in 1851. Even finding rooms to set up her office was a struggle. In her biography of Blackwell, Ishbel Ross wrote,

> She had only to mention her profession to have doors banged in her face.
> This was the age of abortionists, mesmerists, clairvoyants, spiritualists, and quacks of one sort or another. Even Elizabeth's dignity could not overcome the prejudice she encountered....[13]

But she finally found rooms for her office and living space. She announced the opening of her office in the *Tribune* and awaited her patients. Also, as Ross continued,

> She set to work at once to establish relations with the medical profession. It was not her intention to stand aloof as a woman physician; she hoped to become a useful part of the existing medical framework. But here, too, she ran head on into a wall of ice....When she sought permission to visit the women's ward of a city hospital, her application was considered unworthy of notice.[14]

Blackwell wrote of those early days,

The first seven years of New York life were years of very difficult, though steady, work. It was carried on without cessation and without change from town, either summer or winter. I took rooms in University Place, but patients came very slowly to consult me. I had no medical companionship, the profession stood aloof, and society was distrustful of the innovation. Insolent letters occasonally came by post, and my pecuniary position was a source of constant anxiety.

Soon after settling down I made an application to be received as one of the physicians in the women's department of a large city dispensary; but the application was refused, and I was advised to form my own dispensary.[15]

After a very slow year in private practice she again applied for a dispensary position, but was rejected on the grounds that a woman physician would be counterproductive to the harmony of the institution. So, she followed the caustic advice given her and she opened a small infirmary in 1853. Her purpose was stated in the *First Annual Report of the New York Dispensary for Poor Women and Children, 1885.*

The design of this institution is to give to poor women an opportunity of consulting physicians of their own sex. The existing charities of our city regard the employment of women as physicians as an experiment, the success of which has not been sufficiently proven to admit of cordial cooperation. It was therefore necessary to form a separate institution which should furnish to poor women the medical aid which they could not obtain elsewhere....

The Eleventh Ward was chosen as the location for the dispensary, it being destitute of medical charity, while possessing a densely crowded poor population....Over 200 poor women received medical aid. All these women have gratefully acknowledged the help afforded them, and several of the most destitute have tendered their few pence as an offering to the institution.[16]

It is an embarrassment to read of the struggles she withstood: malicious letters, anonymous hate mail, slander from passersby on the street. Yet, she persisted and the number of patients steadily increased. In 1856 she was joined by her sister, Emily, a recent graduate of Rush Medical College, and Marie Zakrzewska, a recent graduate from Western Reserve University with an impressive history in midwifery. In May of 1857 there was an official opening of the Infirmary with its three female physicians.

The Civil War interrupted their plans for establishing a medical college for women, but, Blackwell wrote, "In 1865 the trustees of the infirmary, finding that the institution was established in public favour, applied to the Legislature for a charter conferring college powers upon it."[17] This move was opposed by some of the women physicians associated with the infirmary; they thought that women should have the benefit of training in the larger schools with men. However, the unanimous denial of admission to women convinced all that a separate school was necessary. One of the strong points of the new school, opened officially in 1868, was an Examination Board that set standards higher than existing schools, assuring the quality of the coming generation of women physicians. The school grew steadily and numbered among its faculty, not only the Blackwell sisters and Marie Zakrzewska (who went to Boston and founded the New England Hospital for Women and Children in 1862), but also Mary Putnam Jacobi and Rebecca Cole, the first black woman physician in the United States. Elizabeth Blackwell was appointed Professor of Hygiene. In 1900 the medical college merged with Cornell which now accepted women into its medical school.

The Hygienist

In 1852, the first year of her almost non-existent medical practice, Blackwell used her free time to write a series of six lectures that she delivered in the basement lecture room of Hope Chapel. These lectures were later published as *The Laws of Life with Special Reference to the Physical Education of Girls.* It is difficult for us today to imagine the poverty, filth, and overcrowding of the slums of New York City during the years of massive immigration. The work of John H. Griscom, M.D., and the documentation by Jacob Riis in his 1890 conscience-awakening book, *How the Other Half Lives,* testify to the horrors of the slums. In the lectures Blackwell focused her remarks on women, describing their travails in the society of that day: early marriage and frequent pregnancies, ignorance of health and bodily functions, and no path open to the development of intellectual or other skills. As Ishbel Ross noted,

> She took up one vitiation after another - crowded living conditions, poor ventilation, outmoded Dutch frame houses, unwholesome food, immorality in boarding schools, overcrowded classrooms, overheating by stoves, the disappearance of city gardens, the absence of public squares, the lack of

exercise and sunshine, the decline of religious influence in the home, and various other dilapidations of the fifties.[18]

The second half of the nineteenth century were years of developing reforms in America, a time when there were growing concerns about women's suffrage, temperance, the health of the poor, education, child labor, and other obvious disadvantages present in a country that was entering its Gilded Age of industrial prosperity. Here, again, there is the coexistence of forces driving toward reform of perceived social ills and equally strong economic forces resisting change. Industrialists favored unlimited immigration to meet their need for cheap labor; public health officials and public educators were distressed by what they saw in the slums. Feminism was gathering strength even as it was strongly resisted by men in professions, in clubs, and in courts of law. In this context Blackwell was uniquely placed - both socially and personally - to respond in her special way to what she saw in the city.

One of the more confusing aspects of the Victorian Age is found in comparing the moralisms of those years with rampant prostitution. This was a social evil often addressed by Blackwell. She wrote of the parliamentary documentation of 'white slavery' and the buying and selling of women and children in the United States, England, and France. In an effort to galvanize protection services Blackwell pointed out in a 1879 pamphlet, *Wrong and Right Methods of Dealing with Social Evil,* the differences between the wording of the law, and its actual function.

> In the great majority of the subjects of legislation, the nature and the interests of the two sexes are identical; but the fact of natural difference between men and women...renders it impossible for either sex alone to understand the true aspect of this ineradicable difference, on which just and wise action must be based....
>   The fundamental error of one sex can govern the several relations of both, is a corrupting fallacy,...[19]

Sexual immorality and the failure of both church and state to confront the blatant damage done to women remained a defining concern of this doctor. Abraham Jacobi, the 'Father of American pediatrics,' said of Blackwell in his memorial address in 1911,

> Her lifelong interest in the health of the race was displayed in the attention she paid constantly to the education of the young and adolescent in *sexual questions*....She spoke of these things openly, when our hypocrisy disallowed any discussion of the subject.[20]

Essential to understanding her interest in hygiene is recalling her family background and what little we know of her own personality. She was raised in a religious tradition that had its roots in Puritanism with its strong emphases, not only on morality, but also on intellectual performance. In an address given in October 1889 at the opening of the winter session of the London School of Medicine for Women, Blackwell said,

> With sound intellectual growth, the range of moral influence increases. But such sound growth can only take place under the guidance of moral principle; for moral perception becomes reason, as the intellectual faculties grow; and reason is the true light for all. It is in this high moral life, enlarged by intelligence, that the ideal of womanhood lies.[21]

Blackwell also wrote of her own difficulties with her sexuality and her search for other expressions for that powerful drive that is common human experience. Religion, art, political and social reform, and science are avenues that we can travel down that absorb the energies we sense in the intensities of sexuality and interpersonal relations. In this last half of the nineteenth century reform became a powerful tool for expressing the growing feminist movement. A significant part of this movement was a conviction that prevention was the key to a healthy society. Clean air and water, nutritious food, and a moral (and, coincidently, religious) foundation for society would result in health - both personal and social. To this end, Blackwell developed a corps of sanitary visitors who went into the slums to teach clean habits with their soaps and sponges, clean linens and scrub brushes. Pamphlets describing good health habits were distributed and, when necessary, read to the illiterate. Temperance and chastity, cleanliness and exercise, were pathways to health and wholeness.

Another cause that Blackwell supported was antivivisection. It is important to recall that, in the earlier years of the nineteenth century in England, Scotland and France, anatomy and physiology were taught by dissecting live animals without anesthesia. One wonders about the reactions of observers in those days. Blackwell was alarmed by this method of teaching by animal experimentation, and her argument has a compelling ring to it even today. She wrote,

> Now, the natural instinct to be cherished in human beings is protection and kindliness to infancy and all helpless creatures, not indifference to suffering or wilful infliction of it. As human conscience is a thing of growth or degradation, the natural shrinking from needless pain can soon be hardened into callousness. Conversing with medical students in relation

to the effect made upon them by witnessing vivisections even under chloroform, I have found their experience is always the same - viz., first the shock of repulsion, then tolerance, and then, if often repeated, indifference.[22]

Blackwell's concerns about the uses of animals in research are valid today. She understood Darwin's theory of the origin of our species as a proof of our eternal tie to all the other animals in the creation. The testing of cosmetics in rabbits' eyes, the use of animals by the U.S. Army to study the effects of bullets fired from rifles, hunting and fishing practices, and other examples raise concerns about our indifference to the sufferings of animals. Blackwell also correlated animal dissection with the possibility of the doctor becoming hardened to some patients. She wrote that vivisection

tends to make us less scrupulous in our treatment of the sick and helpless poor. It increases that disposition to regard the poor as 'clinical material,' which has become, alas! not without reason, a widespread reproach to many of the young mentors of our most honorable and merciful profession.[23]

In her strong belief in the primary health functions of personal hygiene and public sanitation, Blackwell took a dim view of the developing science of bacteriology. She saw this new discipline, with what seemed to her to be an apparent detachment from the personal care of patients, as a 'male' profession that would increase the distance between doctor and patient, lessening the healing power of compassion. Bacteriology and the other laboratory sciences appeared to her to distract the physician from concern for the sick. A factor in her attitude was certainly a bitter personal experience that she had when she was deeply shocked by the death of a child whom she had vaccinated against smallpox. An experience like that, as we know, can have a profound impact on our thinking, irrational though it be. She wrote,

The most painful experience which I met with in practice was the death of one of my little patients from the effects of vaccination. This baby, though carefully tended and the lymph guaranteed pure, died....To a hygienic physician thoroughly believing in the beneficence of Nature's laws, to have caused the death of a child by such means was a tremendous blow![24]

Blackwell opted for hygienist as the proper role for the physician. The potential benefits for health and for medical care to be found in the scientific advances that followed the work of Pasteur and Koch's discovery of the tubercle bacillus were lost to her. This obtuse understanding is difficult to meld with the reformists' overarching concern for sanitation: clean water and air. But the concept of invisible organisms causing disease through the media of water, food, and air was difficult to fathom for many in her generation, both physicians and laity.

Commentary

Elizabeth Blackwell, while best known as the first woman to receive an M.D. in the United States, also offers us a picture of a woman who understood herself. In a letter to Marie Zakrzewska she wrote,

> I work chiefly in principles, and you in putting them to practical use; and one is essential to the other in this complex life of ours. You are a natural doctor,...you know I am different from you in not being a natural doctor:...I am never without some patients, but my thought, and active interest, is chiefly given to some of those moral ends, for which I took up the study of medicine.[25]

Blackwell can be criticized for not realizing - or even imagining - the amazing prospects for the new and developing sciences of bacteriology and physiology. But she was not alone, for the value of the germ theory for the therapeutics of medical practice was questioned. John Harley Warner, in his 1986 book, *The Therapeutic Perspective,* wrote,

> Through the mid-1880s bacteriology's explanatory power was in itself insufficient incentive for most American physicians to consider bacteriological knowledge worthwhile for the therapeutic task. Whether or not its etiological pretensions were true was not really the main issue. For the practitioner a central question by which bacteriology's bid for medical attention should be judged was, What practical difference does it make for healing patients?[26]

Blackwell, in her insistence upon hygiene and preventive medicine, is instructive for us today. Certainly, the persistent development of strains of bacteria resistant to antibiotics, the mutation potential of lethal viruses, and the obvious relationships between personal behavior and disease are reminders of the critical need for public health practices and education.

I have noted here the division between the feminist reform movement with its insistence upon the female role as sympathetic caregiver modeled upon the maternal role of wife and mother, and the new sciences which set aside gender as a determinant of profession. Marie Zakrzewska presented the opposing argument in her address to the incoming students of the New England Female Medical College in Boston in 1859.

> However absolutely necessary a certain amount of sympathy and compassion may be, to qualify the physician for success in practice, it will never be the right motive from which the student must start. This predominating, sentimentalizing sympathy will dwarf or confuse the reason...and will be pernicious to logic.[27]

Apparently, both the scientific basis of the profession and its requirement for compassion are needed to produce the good doctor.

But the central lesson for us today is Blackwell's setting of a moral foundation for medicine. She, for reasons stemming from her childhood and adolescence, saw the profession as a moral one, a way of being with, and for, others. Morantz-Sanchez described Blackwell's concern for morality as the basis for medical practice.

> Women physicians, she argued, must monitor medical progress so that it does not violate moral truth. "Whatever revolts our moral sense as earnest women," she reminded her students, "is not in accordance with steady progress" and "cannot be permanently true." It was through the "moral, guiding the intellectual" that the "beneficial influence of women in any new sphere of activity" would be felt.[28]

Elizabeth Blackwell lived and acted in her professional life in ways that anticipated contemporary concerns for 'treating the whole patient.' Not only the physical complaint, but the milieu in which the person lives and functions are factors to be evaluated. She wrote that the exceptional impact that doctors have

> is not only due to the great importance of dealing with the issues of life and death in health and disease, but it is still more owing to the fact that the body and the mind are so inseparably blended in the human constitution, that we cannot deal with the one portion of this compound nature without in more or less degree affecting the other. Our ministrations to the body and soul cannot be separated by a sharply-defined line. The arbitrary distinction between the physician of the body and the physician of the soul - doctor and priest - tends to disappear as science advances.[29]

[1]Roth, Laurence G., "Elizabeth Blackwell - 1821-1910," *Yale Journal of Biology and Medicine,* 20:1, 1947, 3.

[2]Blackwell, Elizabeth, *Pioneer Work in Opening the Medical Profession to Women* (Longmans, 1895), Everyman's Library, New York, E. P. Dutton & Co., Inc., 1914, 21-23.

[3]Ibid., 27-28.

[4]Ibid., 52.

[5]Smith, Stephen, "A Woman Student in a Medical College," *In Memory of Dr. Elizabeth Blackwell and Dr. Emily Blackwell,* New York, Knickerbocker Press, 1911, 3-4.

[6]Ross, Ishbel, *Child of Destiny,* New York, Harper & Brothers, 1949, 114.

[7]Blackwell, *Pioneer..., op.cit.,* Appendix II, 261.

[8]Ibid., 92.

[9]Ibid., 100.

[10]Welch, William H., *In Memory of Dr. Elizabeth Blackwell..., op. cit.,* 51.

[11]Morantz-Sanchez, Regina Markell, *Sympathy and Science,* New York, Oxford University Press, 1985, 4.

[12]Drachman, Virginia G., *Women Doctors and the Women's Medical Movement: Feminism and Medicine, 1850-1895,* State University of New York at Buffalo 1976 Ph.D. Thesis, Ann Arbor, Xerox University Microfilms, 218.

[13]Ross, *op. cit.,* 170.

[14]Ross, Ibid., 171.

[15]Blackwell, *Pioneer..., op. cit.,* 154.

[16]Ibid., 234-235.

[17]Ibid., 191.

[18]Ross, *op. cit.,* 173.

[19]Blackwell, Elizabeth, *Wrong and Right Methods of Dealing with Social Evil,* New York, A. Brentano & Co., 1879, 6.

[20]Jacobi, Abraham, *In Memory of Dr. Elizabeth Blackwell,...op. cit.,* 74-75.

[21]Blackwell, Elizabeth, *The influence of Women in the Profession of Medicine,* Baltimore, 1890, 8-9.

[22]Blackwell, Elizabeth, *Essays in Medical Sociology,* vol. I, London, Ernest Bell, 1902, 112.

[23]Ibid., 43.

[24]Blackwell, *Pioneer..., op. ct.,* 193.

[25]Ross, *op. cit.,* 218.

[26]Harley, John Warner, *The Therapeutic Perspective,* Princeton, Princeton University Press, 1997, 279.

[27]More, Ellen Singer, "'Empathy' Enters the Profession of Medicine," in *The Empathic Practitioner,* edited by Ellen Singer More and Maureen A. Milligan, New Brunswick, NJ, Rutgers University Press, 1994, 25.

[28]Morantz-Sanchez, *op. cit.,* 190-191.

[29]Blackwell, *Essays...,* vol. II, 5-6.

Chapter 9

William Henry Holcombe, 1825-1893

William H. Holcombe, M.D. lived a professional and personal life that invites - I think it even demands - careful study. He lived in the latter two-thirds of the nineteenth century, a time in American history of massive societal change that involved all aspects of personal and social life. His responses to these changes, responses that appear to be contradictory at times, can inform us today. Moshe E. Usadi, in his 1995 thesis for the degree of master in the Department of History at the University of North Carolina, *The Homoeopathic Practice of a Nineteenth Century Southern Physician,* wrote,

> We do not do justice to Holcombe's medical, theological and social alignments and realignments when we perceive them solely as expressions of professional or institutional identity. We achieve a greater understanding of this individual when we see his flight from traditional institutions as part of a personal quest that was familiar to many Americans struggling with the tensions between profession and calling, theory and experience, medical philosophy and medical practice; Holcombe's goal was not to detach himself from his profession or society, but to redefine his relationship with them.[1]

Holcombe challenged a number of commonly accepted social and political beliefs; in his search to find his own place in his profession and in the social order we can see some of the issues competing for allegiance in his time.

Early Years

Holcombe was born in Lynchburg, Virginia in 1825, one of six sons. His father was a physician, a graduate of the University of Pennsylvania Medical School. His mother and father were considered to be part of the Virginia aristocracy. Several years before William was born, they left the Presbyterian church and became Methodists. Apparently, the free will beliefs of this denomination with its emphasis upon democratic principles and a conviction that we can, by our own actions, make ourselves better and therefore more acceptable to God, were definitive of the home in which Holcombe was raised.

Concerns of the parents about Southern slavery, and their commitment to abolition precipitated the move of the family to Indiana in 1842. The father resumed his medical practice and became a Methodist preacher, a combined career that he continued to enjoy. He considered medicine his vocation, but responded also to his call to preach. This combination of medicine and ministry has a long history in America, going back to colonial times, when it was acceptable for other educated members of society - ministers and magistrates - to treat common diseases. Botanical and organic therapies were common knowledge. As I described earlier, Cotton Mather was probably one of the best known 'practicing' ministers. As a young man he had wavered between medicine and ministry as his career; he maintained an ongoing interest in both science and theology, and in later life he was a member of the Royal Society. In his time Boston had only one physician with an M.D. degree, so Mather's knowledge and skills and contacts with England were in demand.

Holcombe followed in his father's footsteps and, in 1847, graduated from the University of Pennsylvania Medical School. He joined his father in practice in Indiana, but then moved to Cincinnati and, in 1852 he relocated in Natchez, Mississippi where he practiced for a decade or so. Following the Civil War he moved to New Orleans where he died in 1893.

Two important decisions were to influence his life and his practice of medicine. The first was his acceptance of homeopathy as his mode of medical practice. The second was his conversion to the religious philosophy of Emanuel Swedenborg. Holcombe's interpretations and applications of these two belief systems defined him, both as a person and as a physician, and will be discussed below. Of equal interest are the interpretations of these choices from the perspective of a father-son relationship. Holcombe chose three positions as defining of himself that were exactly the opposites of his father's convinced beliefs: 1), he became a committed supporter of slavery; 2), he became a convert to homeopathy, convinced that this method of medical practice would replace traditional medicine, labeled allopathy by this new sect; 3), he abandoned the Methodism of his earlier years for the strange and idiosyncratic belief system of Swedenborg. It seems very possible that these choices, viewed within a Freudian perspective, were choices that separated him from his father and established his own identity as an individual. There is no way to verify this opinion of the relationship between father and son. Three themes central to their self-definition were polarized by these two men: 1), their passionate need for a religious commitment that expressed emotion and not just intellectual understanding; 2), a firm stand on the most pressing social issue of the day - slavery; 3), interesting speculation around the defense of, and the attack on, orthodox medical practice.

The Conversion to Homeopathy

By the time Holcombe had moved from Cincinnati to Natchez Homeopathy was well established as a medical sect in America. Its first practitioner, Hans B. Gram, was a Danish immigrant who started his practice in New York City in 1825. His disciple, John F. Gray, opened his office in New York three years later. This unorthodox medical sect had its origins in the work of Samuel Christian Hahnemann (1755-1843), a German physician and theorist. Hahnemann translated *Materia Medica,* the text of the Edinburgh physician, William Cullen, that set forth the theory and practice of bloodletting. Hahnemann, reading Cullen's explanation of the action of cinchona bark on the stomach, decided to study the effects of this drug on himself. He was satisfied by this study that Cullen was wrong. Out of this self-experiment came the first of the three principles of Hahnemann, that of *similia similibus curantur,* 'like cures like.' He had no confidence in the healing power of Nature. The second principle of Hahnemann, based upon his experiment with quinine was the efficacy of minute doses of drugs that, in larger quantities, cause the same symptoms as the disease in question. The third principle was that some seven-eights of all chronic diseases are caused by an infectious disorder called, *Psora,* or the Itch. This was never clearly defined. Hahnemann focused his thought and his practice on the symptoms that patients presented, reasoning that symptoms - not diseases - were the complaints to be treated. From his personal experience with cinchona bark he discerned that symptoms could be alleviated by using medicines that produced similar symptoms in healthy persons, but that they should be given in infinitesimally small doses. A central thesis in his argument was a belief in the old theory of vitalism; out of these thoughts developed an entire medical system that proliferated. Martin Kaufman, in his 1971 book, *Homeopathy in America*, noted the early growth of this sect.

When Hahnemann's works were translated into English and became better known, in the early 1840's, the system gained both in numbers and influence. Its success in the cholera epidemic from 1848 to 1852 brought added publicity and respectability. It was reported that a great many orthodox practitioners were disappointed with the limited success of their own practices in the face of the cholera outbreak. This led to what one historian described as "a widespread desertion from orthodox ranks...."

By the mid-nineteenth century, the new sect had established medical societies in state after state, and in 1844 the American Institute of Homeopathy was organized as the first national medical society. In addition, homeopathic colleges were being founded to train second generation homeopaths. Before 1869, however, the majority of its practitioners were still orthodox physicians who had abandoned their system in favor of the safer and seemingly more effective Hahnemannian method.[2]

The middle years of the nineteenth century saw major changes in how Americans understood themselves, both as a nation and as individuals. Medicine, in particular, seemed to provide a living example of these changes, and homeopathy was important in their persistence. Orthodox physicians, holding to the precepts of Rush and Cullen, supported with vigor the practices of bloodletting and purging as definitive of the properly trained doctor: the hallmarks of orthodoxy. These therapies confirmed for the orthodox the legitimacy of their education and training. There were obvious objections to orthodoxy: 1), public discontent with these practices; 2), the apparently effective appearance of eclectics, hydropaths, and Thomsonians; 3), Jacksonian democratic impulses; and 4), the emergence of the new sciences of physiology and pathology (following upon Paris School and German university influences). All these factors created an atmosphere that welcomed the gentleness and the intellectual dogma of homeopathy. Another aspect of this time of change was the realization that no therapy was often the preferred method of choice in diseases that were self-limited, and in which the body (also read as Nature) was the healer.

The awareness of the value of homeopathic practices in the care of the sick had a specific effect on medical practice in general. As John Harley Warner noted,

The example of homeopathic success showed regular practitioners that often cure could be effected with very mild therapeutic intervention. The recovery of patients under homeopathic care did not necessarily mean that homeopathy actively cured patients - most regular physicians, indeed, regarded the prescription of infinitesimal doses as tantamount to doing nothing; but it did demonstrate that cure often owed more to the healing power of nature than to medical art. As important, the assault upon allopathic therapy incited a popular outcry against heroic drugging; and in a competitive market, regular physicians made their therapies increasingly milder.[3]

Oliver Wendell Holmes delivered two long lectures (some 150 pages in print!) in 1842 titled, "Homoeopathy and its Kindred Delusions." In these lectures he dissected out the apparent and profound errors of the method. In his very sharp and stinging way - noted above in the essay on him - Holmes referred to the science of Homeopathy as

A mingled mass of perverse ingenuity, of tinsel erudition, of imbecile credulity, and of artful misrepresentation, too often mingled in practice, if we may trust the authority of its founder, with heartless and shameless imposition.[4]

The struggles in the nineteenth century with attempts to define what medical practice was - and should be - are intriguing. It is always a challenge to try to understand the complexities of the past, some of which hold over to the present. An article in the eminent British medical journal, *The Lancet,* in 1994 reported on three placebo-controlled studies of the treatment of asthma with oral homeopathic immunotherapy. The results supported the efficacy of homeopathic treatment. The authors, aware of orthodox medical opinion, noted,

The usual response to the possibility that action - asking "how?" before asking "if?" is a bad basis for good science when dealing empirically with things that may as yet evade explanation....Our results lead us to conclude that homeopathy differs from placebo in an inexplicable but reproducible way.[5]

In the nineteenth century regular practitioners argued that, while homeopathic successes merited attention as correctives of the older heroic therapies, the tendency to systematize ran counter to the new scientific methods that were becoming ideals for the proper practice of medicine. Formulaic reasoning also ran counter to the old - yet revered - tradition of attending to the specifics of the patient's story. No two persons were the same and each needed to be treated as an individual with observations dutifully recorded about details of heredity, season, climate, and other factors contributing to the patient's disease and the specific therapy required.

An engaging aspect of the professional life of Holcombe is his rejection of strict adherence to any dogmatic reading of homeopathy or allopathy. In his 1874 pamphlet, *What is Homeopathy?,* he insisted on considering all possible means of helping his patients. He wrote that, when confronted by a patient with a strange or incurable disease for which no homeopathic remedy is known, the physician should not retire from the struggle. Is he to give them up...? Not if he is a man of scientific culture and independent character. He will do the best he can under the circumstances. He will palliate by every means in his power; and it is astonishing sometimes what relief homeopathic remedies can give, even when they cannot cure. But he need not confine himself to homeopathic remedies. *His treatment should be empirical - anything and everything which promises to do his patient any good. If he falls short here of the most intelligent and wide-extended eclecticism, he is ignorant of his duty or faithless to his trust.*[6]

This placement of the needs of the patient before any sectarian rule-of-thumb is a very impressive part of the personality of Holcombe, adding to an understanding of him as an 'eclectic' in more ways than medical.

Another influence of homeopathy was the challenge to heroic therapy offered by women physicians. The attributes of femininity were easily translated into offering kinder care, especially to women and children, than the traditional treatments prescribed by men. Regina Morantz-Sanchez, writing in 1997, noting that "Many women physicians did spurn heroic medicine," quoted from a biographical sketch of Hannah Longshore:

[M]any intelligent women had become tinctured with the heresy of Homeopathy and gave a preference to the physician who would prescribe or administer their milder and pleasant remedies,...This discovery led the woman doctor to an investigation of their remedies and theories of therapeutics and to partial adoption of their remedies and methods of treatment.[7]

This method of adapting new therapies to fit experience is the same as the one used by Holcombe, only in reverse: he used the Hahnemann system to the extent that it suited the needs of his patients as interpreted by him through his learning in his general medical education.

One of the delights in the story of Holcombe's medical career is his personalized approach to his chosen profession of medicine. He struggled to bring together in his own person his social convictions, his medical experiences, and his spiritual beliefs. As Usadi noted in his thesis on Holcombe,

He assimilated bits and pieces of the ideas and values of a wide variety of individuals around him in order to create a unique personal philosophy....Medicine formed the cornerstone of Holcombe's personal philosophy because it allowed him to interact with his community in a concrete way even though his personal reality differed from the reality of most of those around him. But his profession also caused Holcombe a great deal of frustration because the ignorance and materialism of those he served debased what he believed to be in essence a noble profession.[8]

Holcombe was certainly concerned about his success as a practitioner, but that concern was sharply defined by his personal commitments to his community and to his religious faith, a faith that was as new - and to many observers as strange - as homeopathy in America.

The New Churchman

At some time in his early professional life, Holcombe came in contact with the writings of Emanuel Swedenborg (1688-1772), an amazing combination of Christian mystic, scientist, theologian, and philosopher. At the age of 27 Swedenborg was the publisher of Sweden's first scientific journal, including in it results of his own studies and projects. He was appointed assessor of the Royal Mines, devoting himself to their improvement for thirty years. During that time he developed a theory of invisible particles and of the nature of the solar system that is amazingly close to our contemporary thought. In his sixties he made extensive and accurate studies of anatomy, in particular of the brain and of the circulation. He was the author of some thirty books.

At this same period in his life Swedenborg underwent a painful religious crisis. Developing from a number of dreams and visions of Christ - both in his dreams and while awake - Swedenborg came to the realization that there was an identification between the power of God and the presence of God in all that lives. The 1992 edition of *the Encyclopedia Britannica* describes his thought thusly:

> In his theology he asserts the absolute unity of God....The Father, Son, and the Holy Spirit represent a trinity of essential qualities of God: love, wisdom, and activity. This divine trinity is reproduced in human beings in the form of the trinity of soul, body, and mind....Swedenborg attempted to interpret the Scriptures in the light of the "correspondence" between the spiritual and material planes. He viewed references in the Bible to mundane historical matters as symbolically communicating spiritual truths, the key to which he tried to find through detailed and voluminous commentaries and interpretations.[9]

One can see the liberating force to a physician of this concept of the presence of God in all of life. Swedenborg believed that his writings would provide the foundation for what he called a "New Church." And he was correct; the first new church was established the year of his death, 1788, and the General Conference of the New Church (England) continues to meet to this day. The first American society was organized in Baltimore in 1792; there are now two colleges in the United States that offer four-year courses for ordination.

A concern much in the mind of Holcombe was the similarity in thought between the Transcendentalists of New England and the non-traditional ideas of Swedenborg. Holcombe was an admirer of the writings of Emerson, but not of the Puritan background that Holcombe saw behind them. There was a freeing sensation to be known in the conviction that God is present at all times and in all places and that there are higher laws that govern our lives and our created universe. There was also a freedom from the ancient liturgy and routine celebrations, a freedom that opened up a world of sensibility and spontaneity to the New Churchman, as it did for the New England innovative thinkers and writers. The sense of a spirituality potentially present to all persons was an invigorating force for both Northern Transcendentalists and Southern Intellectuals. There was also a persistent and strong hold-over in America of the ideas of the Enlightenment that supported a willingness to admit of many and varied paths to the Truth. One of the examples of this was widespread sectarianism, both in medicine and in religion, two of Holcombe's concerns. Usadi commented in his thesis that,

> It is appropriate that the language of faith and the language of science were linked in discussions of homeopathy, as they were in discussions of other medical traditions as well, for theology and science were related topics during the nineteenth century. This was also a period of sectarian conflict in the United States when proponents of competing religious traditions argued about the proper means of saving souls and serving God, while supporters of different therapeutic schools clashed over the best means of curing the body and serving society.[10]

Holcombe was amazingly talented in his ability to hold his New Churchman stance and his commitment to homeopathy together and build a successful practice based upon integrity and his openness to new ideas and principles. Moving to Natchez, Mississippi in 1852 he joined another homeopathic physician, F.A.W. Davis, both in private practice and as physician to the Mississippi State Hospital. Holcombe was impressive as a person who tried to view all the patients in his practice as individuals in a society that required medical care. He allowed experience to temper his theories of disease and of treatment.

The Slavery Issue

Although there were impressive similarities in the thoughts and writings of the New England Transcendentalists and the Southern Intellectuals, their sharp conflict over slavery created a dividing line not to be crossed. At first it seems inconceivable that a competent and caring physician, an educated man committed to a novel, yet demanding, religious faith could support the institution of slavery. Aside from the imagined father-son psychological conflict projected earlier, it turns out that the mystical nature of the religious construct proposed by Swedenborg fitted well into a justification for human slavery as it existed in the United States. Repugnant as his views are today, they must be interpreted and understood in the context of the time.

In 1861 Holcombe published a pamphlet, *Suggestions as to the Spiritual Philosophy of African Slavery Addressed to the Members and Friends of the Church of the New Jerusalem.* The theological framework is convoluted and highly imagined, even to a level of fantasy. The "African races" and "our Indian aborigines" are descendants of persons who lived before the Flood, labeled by Swedenborg as being of a *celestial* type. Proof of this lies, according to Holcombe, in the African's "ineradicable childishness, - his light-heartedness, simplicity, credulity, and timidity, - in his passion for music and dancing, in his forgiving temper, and in that beautiful willingness to serve,..."[11] Holcombe continued with a discussion of the relationships between skin color - red and black - and "perversions of charity and truth" that survived the nearly complete destruction of all living things in the Flood.

Holcombe stressed his very strong objections to slavery when it occurred within the same race: whites enslaved by whites and Africans enslaved by Africans. There was a reason for African slaves being brought into obedience and subjection by white men:

> The white man *wills* and *thinks* for him, determines his outgoings and his incomings, his food, his clothing, his sleep, his work, etc. He compels him to do uses under a rational and scientific supervision. He makes him obedient as a child, partly by affectionate control, partly by fear of corporeal punishment.[12]

The result of this relationship is the development of a truthful, virtuous, and affectionate African man. Holcombe made the point that the African can never become what the white man is. "The Negro is a child - not to be made a man of our sort by any amount of political or scientific culture. The relation of master and slave is for him a far better and happier one than that of capitalist and laborer."[13]

Holcombe was convinced that the African slave had achieved a far higher level of development under Southern guidance than would be possible elsewhere. He suggested that Southern masters would become abolitionists if there was any evidence that Africans, considering their inherent nature and capacities, would do better in a different environment. Holcombe closed his pamphlet with the observation that the developing spiritual life of the universe would confirm the blessings of slavery.

> [N]ot only is his slaveholding not a sin, but it is a blessing to all around him,...The unfolding of the spiritual world may possibly reveal the fact, that this Christian slaveholder, misunderstood and reviled as he now is by his brethren in other countries, has attained the sublimest point of human civilization.[14]

Commentary

Holcombe presents us with a challenge: how do we understand a man with strong commitments to the care of his patients, a man with a religious faith that he showed forth in his medical practice and his relationships, and a man convinced of the logic and necessity of human slavery? This question has been an ongoing one in studies of American slavery; Thomas Jefferson being an outstanding enigma in this issue. The existence of slavery in varied forms throughout our history, including the enslavement of Africans by Africans who would then provide the slaves who were abducted and bought, is an odd and very disturbing part of our human record. As I noted, Holcombe and many other Southern Intellectuals were comfortable with the practice that he defended. We are left with the contradiction of a man dedicated to the care of all persons even if it involved sacrifice on the part of the doctor, and a man convinced of the rightness of slavery.

Holcombe was alert to the powerful impact of the mind on the body, an emerging awareness among physicians in that time. He believed this to the extent of his conviction that fear is an accepted cause of medical diseases. In an Appendix to a 1898 book, *Happiness as Found in Forethought minus Fearthought,* by Horace Fletcher, Holcombe noted the relationship between fear and yellow fever.

[T]he subjects connected with the disease are strongly pictured on the mind. They are talked of, read about, discussed and written about, until the mind is full of images of fever, delirium, black vomit, jaundice, death, funerals, etc. When such is the case, no microbes or bacteria are needed to produce an outburst of yellow fever. The whole mass of horrors already stamped upon the mind is simply reflected and repeated in the body.[15]

Holcombe achieved success in his profession; he was successful in his practice and also was elected president of the American Institute of Homeopathy in 1875. He made a concerted effort to bring the new profession of homeopathy into accord with the beliefs of established medical doctors. In the concluding statement in his pamphlet, *What is Homoeopathy,* he wrote that

The closer our approximation to the truth on any subject, the more thoroughly we shall agree in opinion....Knowledge is the true and only healer of dissensions. The powerful ferment of thought which characterizes the present century, will eventuate in a better order of things, and the establishment of the true fundamental principles of theology, government, science, and art. For medicine, too, and medical men, there is a coming millennium and the reign of brotherly love.[16]

He was a poet, the author of a novel, and a loyal follower of Emanuel Swedenborg. His religious faith incorporated the Methodist doctrine of a grace that could be achieved by good works with the "church within the church" ideas of Swedenborg to present a physician who apparently lived a moral and admirable life. One of the aspects of his career that is telling is a persistent strain of self-doubt that he noted in his diary, brief as it was. He was the intellectual companion of Emerson and Thoreau, but could not accept their northern characteristics. He was a physician convinced of the centrality of the profession in caring for others, yet he chose a sect of medical practice that was to diminish to insignificance toward the end of his life.

Instructive for the student of medical history is the part of Holcombe's person that steadily sought to learn and that was open to new ideas and to concepts. Another segment of his person was his search for a spiritual and moral basis for his life and his work. The need for a foundation to his life that would determine both his work and his relationships with his world is evident in his story. His search for this foundation is an important reminder for all of us.

In a book of his poems, *Southern Voices,* published in 1872, Holcombe included one called "Free." The reader senses a sea-change in his understanding of the institution of African slavery, so recently ended by the Emancipation Proclamation and the catastrophic Civil War.

YES! we are glad they are free.
Free let them ever remain!
Perish the wrongs of the past!
No curse, no bondage again!
Ring out the bells on the air!
Ring them from mountain to sea!
Ring for the Night which has gone,
And the Day which is to be!
Let the soldier sheathe his sword!
Let the Christian kiss his cross!
And all of us count with joy
The gain we thought was loss!
And the skies will flash with light,
And the hills resound again,
"Glory to God in the highest!
Peace and good-will to men!"[17]

[1]Usadi, Moshe E., *The Homoeopathic Practice of a Nineteenth Century Southern Physician*, Thesis submitted to the faculty of the University of North Carolina at Chapel Hill in partial fulfillment for the degree of master in the Department of History, 1995, 3-4.
[2]Kaufman, Martin, *Homeopathy in America*, The Johns Hopkins Press, Baltimore, 1971, 29.
[3]Warner, John Harley, "Orthodox and Otherness: Homeopathy and Regular Medicine in Nineteenth-Century America," *Culture, Knowledge, and Healing*, ed. R. Jutte, G.B. Risse, J. Woodward, European Association for the History of Medicine and Health Publications, Sheffield, 1998, 8.
[4]Holmes, Oliver Wendell, "Homoeopathy, and its Kindred Delusions," *Currents and Counter-Currents in Medical Science*, Boston, Ticknor and Fields, 1861, 176.
[5]Reilly, D., Taylor, M.A., Beattie, N.G., Campbell, J.H., McSharry, C., Aitchison, T.C., Carter, R., and Stevenson, R.D., "Is evidence for homeopathy reproducible?" *The Lancet*, December 10, 1994, 344:1606.
[6]Holcombe, William H., *What is Homeopathy?*, Boericke & Tafel, New York, 1874, 23-24.
[7]Morantz-Sanchez, Regina, "The 'Connecting Link': The Case for the Woman Doctor in 19th Century America," *Sickness & Health in America*, edited by Leavitt, J.W., and Numbers, R.L., University of Wisconsin Press, Madison, Wisconsin, 1997, 218.

[8]Usadi, *op. cit.,* 34-35.
[9]*The New Encyclopaedia Britannica,* 15th edition, 1992, Chicago, Encylopaedia Britannica, Inc., Volume 11, 438.
[10]Usadi, *op. cit.,* 41.
[11]Holcombe, William H., *Suggestions as to the Spiritual Philosophy of African Slavery Addressed to the Members and Friends of the Church of the New Jerusalem,* New York, Mason Brothers, 1861, 4.
[12]Ibid., 7.
[13]Ibid., 11.
[14]Ibid., 24.
[15]Holcomb(*sic),* Dr. Wm. H., "The Influence of Fear in Disease," in Fletcher, Horace, *Happiness as Found in Forethought minus Fearthought,* Chicago & New York, Herbert S. Stone & Co., 1898, 230-231.
[16]Holcombe, *What is Homeopathy?, op. cit.,* 28.
[17]Holcombe, Wm, H., *Southern Voices: Poems,* Philadelphia, J. B. Lippincott & Co., 1872, 42.

Chapter 10

Mary Putnam Jacobi, 1842-1906

In his Foreword to the 1925 book, *Life and Letters of Mary Putnam Jacobi,* George Haven Putnam wrote these lines about his sister:

> This volume presents a sketch of the life and work of a woman whose personality was assuredly distinctive and who was able, through persistent and capable work, to render noteworthy service to her fellows, service the influence of which will continue through the later generations....Mary Putnam was endowed with vision and imagination, and the things accomplished by her gave evidence of courage and will power, through which some at least of these visions were brought to realization. Her decisions and actions were strongly influenced by sentiment, but she abhorred sentimentality.[1]

For any student of medicine this Victorian Age woman is a stellar example of accomplishment - both personal and professional - in the face of impressive opposition in nineteenth century American medicine. Before reviewing the life and the work of this physician, the social and educational tempers of the times must be evaluated since they were powerful factors in casting the roles of women and men in those years. There was a profound ambivalence about what women should - even could - do in those years of profound change in so many categories of American life. Massive immigration, sharp fluctuations in the economy from boom to bust associated with rapid development of industrialization, and a palpable sense of the need for reforms shook the established order of society. These events introduced, however, possibilities for radical changes. Not the least of these was the growing demand from women for entry into the professions.

An Age of Reform

In the 1830s and 1840s there were dedicated efforts initiated to reform American middle class culture. Education for women became a realizable possibility, and women's suffrage emerged as an issue that would not go away. Part of the growing awareness of personal rights and necessities was the dismay and the distrust that evolved into convinced attitudes that women held toward physicians and their treatment of women. Integral to this growing wariness about male physicians was the obvious fact that men could not *know* what women experienced in their physical lives, particularly their sexual and maternal experiences.

Advances in studies in physiology and chemistry in Europe in the first third of the nineteenth century raised serious questions about the 'heroic' therapies of purging, puking and bleeding so common in America. Unfortunately, with this new knowledge there was no concomitant development of new therapies, leaving a vacuum in therapeutics into which sectarian practitioners moved quickly, sharing the popular discontent and dismay with traditional doctors. The advent of anesthesia called into question the image of the surgeon as a man needing the character and the will of an executioner.

The ways in which middle class women understood themselves and their positions in society underwent a similar upheaval. The rapid growth in industries that followed upon the Civil War created an urban middle class with financial capabilities for servants. This freed these women from laborious household chores of cooking, sewing, and cleaning. This new freedom offered middle class women an opportunity to revalue their lives. There were a number of strong social movements - temperance, suffrage, hygiene, and abolition - that raised religious, moral, and societal concerns to a powerful emotional level. All of this occurred during the years we know as the Victorian Age of corsets, petticoats and full skirts, and very mixed responses to basic human desires and drives. A powerful polarization of gender definition emerged: feminine traits of sympathetic love and maternal caring were combined with a recognition of the supposed reality of the ill-health and limited passionate needs of the weaker sex; men were urged to submit their carnal sexual drives to the wishes of their wives.

These issues offered distinct and difficult choices for many women: to be at home as the perfect wife and mother, supporting the spiritual and moral foundations of the social order; or, setting aside those traditional roles and, using one's intelligence and sensitivity to social needs, entering the real world as a physician, a geologist, or a businesswoman? There were gender differences that were assumed to be irrevocable and timeless, making equality between the sexes in the world outside the home impossible. In a remarkably inventive and imagined paper read before The League for Political Education in 1896, Putnam Jacobi said,

All sorts of causes are constantly forcing women into competition with men,...and then they find themselves under the immense disadvantage of an *a priori* presumption of inferiority....Women have not been excluded from politics, any more than they were, until most recently, forbidden access to learning, because any experiment had shown them incapable, for they had never been put to the test. But they have been counted incapable *because* they have been excluded, through an immemorial tradition, based on considerations with which the question of capacity had nothing to do.[2]

But there were other concerns, especially about women becoming physicians.

Opposition to women entering the medical profession was very strong. Some doctors saw this a threat to their economic security, especially those who treated 'women's diseases.' But there were also strong sentiments voiced about their physical capabilities, their supposed faintheartedness that would certainly appear in anatomy classes, their lack of that unfeeling nature demanded of those who were surgeons and bonesetters. In her contribution to Annie Nathan Meyer's 1891 book, *Woman's Work in America,* Putnam Jacobi effectively quoted from a *Dissertation on Female Physicians* by N. Williams, M.D. that had been read before a New York Medical Society meeting in 1850.

The bare thought of married females engaging in the medical profession is palpably absurd. It carries with it a sense of shame, vulgarity, and disgust. Nature is responsible for my unqualified opposition to educating females for the medical profession.[3]

Dr. Williams's opinion notwithstanding, women in the middle third of the nineteenth century began studying medicine. Because most medical school doors were closed to them, women sought admission to the few women's medical schools extant, entered the numerous sectarian schools, or went abroad to study. In 1849 Elizabeth Blackwell graduated from Geneva Medical College, becoming the first woman to be granted an M.D. in America. The tempest roused by this event caused the school to refuse entry to women thereafter, thanks in part to letters like this one written by D.K. to the *Boston Medical and Surgical Journal* in 1849, a month after Miss Blackwell received her diploma.

The ceremonies of graduating Miss Blackwell at Geneva may be called a farce. I am sorry that Geneva should be the first to commence the nefarious process of amalgamation. The profession was quite too full before.[4]

Sex and Education

In 1873 a member of the Massachusetts Medical Society and Late Professor of Materia Medica at Harvard, Edward H. Clarke, M.D., published a book, *Sex in Education: or a Fair Chance for the Girls.* This book, an expanded version of an address he gave to a meeting of the New-England Women's Club in Boston the year before, called forth powerful responses, *pro* and *contra,* from the public. It was widely read, going into at least five editions. He pointed out that the monthly menstrual cycle was understood as a 'disease' of women; certainly a young woman could go to school and master the material as well as a young man,

> But it is not true that she can do all this, and retain uninjured health and a future secure from neuralgia, uterine disease, hysteria, and other derangements of the nervous system, if she follows the same method that boys are trained in. Boys must study and work in a boy's way, and girls in a girl's way. They may study the same books, and attain an equal result, but should not follow the same method.[5]

Girls needed to prepare for the onset of menstruation, and take appropriate care of their bodies once this monthly event became established. Failure to this could be disastrous, for the *body* cannot do its work appropriately if energies are being directed to the *brain.* Clarke knew patients who "graduated from school or college excellent scholars, but with undeveloped ovaries. Later they married and were sterile. The system never does two things well at the same time. The muscles and the brain cannot *functionate* in their best way at the same moment."[6]   Clarke was definitely in favor of education for both boys and girls: "Appropriate education of the two sexes, carried as far as possible, is a consummation devoutly to be desired: identical education of the two sexes is a crime before God and humanity, that physiology protests against, and that experience weeps over."[7]

The responses to this book were what we would anticipate. It became a physiologically rational support for men who saw the entry of women into medicine as a threat, both to income and to the profession. After all, what woman physician could respond to a medical emergency that might occur during that one week out of every month when she was incapacitated? The book also became a driving force among women eager to disprove this thesis and free themselves from stereotypical roles of housewife, mother, guardian of public morals, and preserver of beauty - personal and cultural. Two alternative approaches to this issue were seen as possible and both were used, providing two distinct models. *First,* the standard attributes of womanhood - kindness, gentleness, compassion, attentive listening - could add immeasurably to the qualities one hoped for in one's doctor. Ellen S. More, in her 1999 book, *Restoring the Balance,* commented on the experiences of women entering medicine.

> I interpret their history as a careful attempt to fulfill expectations that originally were characteristic of mainstream professional culture in nineteenth century medicine....
>
> Although all physicians, male and female, are charged to be both empathic and expert, the historically dichotomous identity imputed to women physicians in Western culture - to be womanly as well as scientific - has complicated the challenge, while situating it at the center of their professional life....Throughout their history, women physicians have attempted to integrate professionalism with civic and personal life,...[8]

This integration of personal and professional roles would be particularly applicable for women who treated women's diseases, eliminating the embarrassment of talking with, and being examined by, a man. A woman's 'natural' empathy toward children would make her an ideal caregiver for them. For many women and men this approach was logical, fitting in with the rapidly growing hygienic movement becoming attractive to middle class women.

A *second* alternative for women was to disregard the obvious gender bias and become a physician trained in the new laboratory sciences of physiology, pathology, chemistry, and bacteriology. While sensitive to the reform tenor of the times, these women were wary of allying their goal of becoming doctors with the sentimentality so easily labeled a feminine characteristic. Accepting the natural gender differences, these women chose not to use them as their reasons for choice of profession. One of these women, to be presented in a subsequent chapter, was Alice Hamilton, who became the first industrial physician in the United States.

An approach that ignored gender and stressed the new sciences taught in superior university medical schools and extended hospital training seemed the better one. A number of women broke the barriers and accomplished successful careers easily equaling, and often surpassing, their male counterparts. One of these women was Mary Putnam Jacobi. At a 1907 convocation of the Women's Medical Association of New York City in memory of Dr. Jacobi, William Osler commented on the struggles of women physicians and on the accomplishments of Jacobi.

Between the open hostility of the many and the half-hearted sympathy of the few, the position of those in the profession was a most unenviable one. That in the past quarter of a century the long battle has been won is due less to a growing tolerance among physicians at large, less to the persistence with which obvious rights have been asserted, than to the presence of a few notable figures who have demonstrated the capacity of women for the highest intellectual development and who have compelled recognition by the character of work accomplished in the science and in the art of medicine.

Among these figures Mary Putnam Jacobi stands prominent.[9]

Mary Putnam Jacobi

Mary Putnam was the eldest child of Victorine Haven and George Palmer Putnam. Both parents traced their families back to seventeenth century Puritan settlers of New England. George Putnam became a major New York publisher - G.P. Putnam & Sons - and an ambivalent supporter of his daughter's career. He held quite strongly to the belief that a daughter's proper place was in the home caring for her parents until a husband was found. Lacking the possibility of a medical education in New York, Mary Putnam studied pharmacy and received a degree from the New York College of Pharmacy in 1863. Still wanting to become a physician, she went to Philadelphia where she attended the Women's Medical College of Pennsylvania for two terms, graduating with her doctor's degree in April 1864. She spent a few months with Dr. Maria Zakrzewska at the New England Hospital for Women and Children, but finally decided that the best opportunities for training were in Paris, and at the age of twenty-four she began studies at the École de Médecine. She would be the second woman to receive a degree from that school, graduating in 1871 with high honors and a bronze medal for her thesis.

Putnam returned to New York and, in 1872, began her decades-long career in teaching at the Woman's Medical College of the New York Infirmary, founded in 1868 by Elizabeth Blackwell. In that year Putnam was elected to membership in the Medical Society of the County of New York. A delightful personal touch: the president of the Medical Society, Abraham Jacobi, welcomed Putnam; indeed, this man, a German-Jewish refugee from the 1848 revolutions in Europe, often referred to as the Father of American Pediatrics became enchanted with her, proposed to her, and they were married in July 1873.

A side note is instructive of the professional environment of the times. As described above, Edward H. Clarke's 1873 book, *Sex in Education,* created an uproar among women. Its clear separation of the academic possibilities for the sexes along physiological lines, especially in relation to menstruation, set the stage for the 1874 announcement by Harvard Medical School of the topic for the Boylston Prize of 1876: the effects of menstruation on women. A group of women in Boston wrote to Putnam Jacobi asking her to win the prize for the cause of women. Putnam did so with her anonymous essay, *The Question of Rest for Women during Menstruation,* much to the later chagrin of male opposition. Her 232 page essay discussed at length a convoluted argument concerning the role of nutrition in menstruation. But she was able to show, by both statistical analyses and case studies, that healthy women functioned fully regardless of their menstrual cycle. Her conclusion was italicized: *"There is nothing in the nature of menstruation to imply the necessity, or even the desirability, of rest, for women whose nutrition is really normal."[10]* After her lengthy presentation, however, she noted that nearly 50% of women suffer during menstruation. Her final words were, "humanity dictates that rest from work during the period of pain be afforded whenever practicable.[11] This essay was the starting point for her remarkable career as teacher, writer, organizer, and clinician.

The Career

Putnam Jacobi practiced medicine while continuing her teaching at the Woman's Medical College. She was offered positions at other schools and hospitals, but chose to stay in New York in an academic environment that she cherished. She wrote nine books, over 120 medical articles, and was a member of the New York Pathological Society, the New York Neurological Society, the New York Academy of Medicine, and founder, in 1874, of what would become The Women's Medical Association. Her professional life encapsulated the best of the ongoing women's movement that pressed for equality in opportunity in the professions. In what could be a summary of the accomplishments of these women in the last quarter of the nineteenth century, we have this excerpt from Putnam Jacobi's chapter, "Woman in Medicine," in Meyer's *Woman's Work in America.*

What women have learned, they have in the main taught themselves. And it is fair to claim, that when they have taught themselves so much, when they have secured the confidence of so many thousand sick persons, in the teeth of such vigorous and insulting opposition, and upon such scanty resources and such inadequate preparation; when such numbers have been able to establish reputable and even lucrative practice, to care for the health of many families over long terms of years,...to restore to health many thousand women who had become helpless invalids from dread of consulting men physicians,...to hold their own in private practice, in matters of judgment, diagnosis, medical and operative treatment, amidst the incessant and often unfair rivalry of brother competitors - to do all this, we repeat, itself demonstrates a very considerable, indeed an unexpected amount of native ability and medical fitness on the part of women.[12]

Putnam Jacobi had, in fact, done all that she described. And she did it with a dedication and energy that amazed others.

Her distress at the poor education of her first students at the Woman's Medical College of the New York Infirmary led to a rapid improvement of their training to help these women face the demands of their futures. She was a major drawing power at the Infirmary, an outstanding attraction for her students. Regina Markell Morantz-Sanchez, in her 1985 book, *Sympathy and Science,* wrote,

"Dr. Jacobi," recalled one of her favorite students, "had an amazing fund of general medical knowledge and was said to be the most widely read medical person in New York City at the time." Although her prolific medical writings were well known and admired, she also excelled as a clinician. "Her knowledge of diagnosis and differential diagnosis was profound," remembered Emily Dunning Barringer, "and based on fundamental understanding of the basic sciences back of medicine. She was a hard taskmaster; there were no short cuts in establishing a diagnosis....What could have been more valuable for an impressionable young doctor just starting out, than to find herself in this atmosphere of truly great scientific accomplishment and to have all her standards of medical procedure crystallized day by day?"[13]

Putnam Jacobi was able to achieve an equality in a profession renowned for its conservative standing on almost all matters. Resistance to admitting women to some medical schools persisted well into the twentieth century.

One of her strong points was her commitment to the sciences as one of the ways to uncovering what we call truth. A strong opponent of 'opinion' in most matters, Putnam Jacobi was an advocate of the library as definer of reality in medical science. One way to understand her impact on medicine and on the entry of women into the profession is to see her in comparison with her colleague of several years, Elizabeth Blackwell, some 21 years her senior. Where Blackwell defined the practice of medicine within her reforming model of hygiene as the way to health, and distrusted the new sciences as barriers to personalized care of the sick, Putnam Jacobi separated science from morality. Morantz-Sanchez commented,

> In her private life she [Jacobi] too confronted the moral dilemmas of the reformer, and she enthusiastically supported meliorist efforts,...But though she understood that the pursuit of truth could never be divorced totally from moral life, she approached the acquisition of medical knowledge as something quite independent of morality. Believing in science with an earnestness that was almost extreme...she viewed scientific research as an absolute good because it added to the fund of human knowledge.[14]

In her Inaugural Address at the opening of the Woman's Medical College of the New York Infirmary in 1880, Putnam Jacobi wrote,

> Many moral qualities are needed in the practice of medicine to meet the difficulties which, though extrinsic to the case considered as an intellectual problem, are very important in its practical discussion....The theoretical and the practical are inextricably intertwined;...

She continued in her Address with a most delightful presentation of the impossibilities associated with any attempt to be a good physician. She wrote,

> You see, therefore, that in order to be a physician, it is not sufficient to have a good memory and be able to pass examinations. This is indispensable, but much more is required. The capacity to examine minutely, yet generalize comprehensively; to take large views, yet not overlook the smallest details; to be quick to notice, yet slow to speak; to reason cautiously, yet decide promptly; to be at once very cool and very warm; to be tenacious of one's reputation, yet indifferent of careless opinions; to be sensitive, yet not touchy; to be patient in temper, yet capable of wrath; to be absolutely honest, yet successfully prudent; to be unworldly, yet capable of managing the forces of the world - all these mental and moral capacities are necessary to enable a physician to study practical medicine, to practice medicine, and to build up a practice out of services rendered to a crowd of sufferers, at once helpless, ignorant, exacting, and capricious. Varied as are the mental and moral capacities required for this enterprise, they may all be traced back to three, namely: Ability to think, character in control, and honor to act from an internal instead of an external standard of obligation.[15]

Commentary

Mary Putnam Jacobi is an outstanding model for all medical students and physicians. There are some aspects of her life - professional and personal - that call us to examine the ends we seek and the means we choose to work toward them. Although she was, as we are, trapped in her own time and place, her approach to making decisions that defined herself are applicable to us today. I shall discuss a few of the defining points of her life.

1. The contributions of women to medicine. Putnam Jacobi instructs us in her refusal to accept any professional definition of herself other than that of a highly trained and skilled physician committed to accurate diagnosis and treatment. In the last quarter of the nineteenth century - a time of severe need for social and political reform - she consistently stressed the need for women to become fully competent in their professions. This would be the only way for them to find their rightful place in society. There was no question that men dominated educational facilities, the professions, and the market place, making access for women difficult. The ethos of the Victorian Age that so widely separated the inherent natures of the two sexes made it difficult for women to break down characterizations of themselves that had long been accepted. In an article, "Shall Women Practice Medicine?" for the January 1882 *North American Review* Putnam Jacobi discussed the need for women to strive for higher occupations, such as the profession of medicine.

> When we shall be rid of the injustice, the unfairness, the monstrous pretensions, and arrogant argument with which the subject of the admission of women to medicine has hitherto been so largely treated; when the mass of women students can obtain the same education and women physicians the same facilities that men do, a sound theoretical conclusion may then be reached, if required.[16]

It would be a while before it would be concluded that women were the equals of men. Removing the barrier of acquiescence to male domination assumed by a superior male intellect was a major task for women who hoped to succeed in achieving the education needed for professional accomplishment.

Putnam Jacobi agreed that women had unique skills in caring for the sick, for children, and for the insane. In a paper delivered at a Social Science Congress in 1881 she showed her commitment to education - especially moral education - in the management of the mentally ill.

There is an amazing modern note to her thinking, taking the time frame of the language into consideration. She wrote,

[T]he three great elements in the moral substratum of a person disposed to insanity, are: the egotistical predominance of the instincts over the faculties of reflection and external relation; the ineffectiveness of the will, even when this is impulsive or violent; the inaptitude for ideas, resulting in their poverty and imperfect combination. The whole nature is shrunken upon itself; there is not enough vital turgescence to expand it to its normal circumference, and to the points of contact of this with the external world.[17]

She agreed that the socially defined skills of women's personalities - empathy and compassion - should not prevent them from entering whichever field of medicine they wished. She deplored the tendency for women to specialize in diseases of women, isolating themselves, not only with their patients, but with other women who made the same choice of specialty. It was important for women to gain a firm foothold in all areas of medicine, including surgery. In essence, she attempted to minimize gender differences so that women would accomplish their goals based upon their abilities, not upon their dependence upon the advice of dominant men.

2. The life of the intellect. This aspect of personality was highly developed in Putnam Jacobi, and one that she stressed to her students and colleagues. Not only was the intellect a pathway to breaking through the barriers erected against women, but also a way of becoming a good doctor in caring for the sick. Morantz-Sanchez wrote,

The respect of her male colleagues was never in doubt. One younger member of the Pathological Society, for example, [Dr. Allan Wyeth] remembered her as a woman "whose knowledge of pathology was so thorough, whose range of the literature was so wide and whose criticism was so keen, fearless and just that in our discussions, we felt it prudent to shun the field of speculation and to walk strictly in the path of demonstrated fact.[18]

One of the ways Putnam Jacobi developed her intellectual life and achieved professional excellence was through writing. She, like many youngsters who are readers, wrote some short pieces about Life when she was between the ages of eight and ten. At age sixteen she had a short story, "Found and Lost," published in the *Atlantic Monthly* for which she received eighty dollars. She pressed her conviction that the study of language was always a primary task for all. At the conclusion of her 1889 book, *Physiological Notes on Primary Education and the Study of Language,* she wrote,

Language which alone perfectly expresses all internal thought, also mirrors all external things as they have ever impressed the mind of man. Language, speech, is thus truly the Logos, the intermediary between the soul and the world. It is at once the thought made flesh and flesh sublimated into thought.[19]

Putnam Jacobi continued to write while she studied in Paris. She became a correspondent for the New York *Evening Post* and began writing articles for the New York *Medical Record;* she continued to submit medical papers of increasing sophistication to this journal for many years. For students today she is a good example of one of the ways to pursue an academic career: write! She wrote articles on many topics, usually based upon case histories, and often with a foundation in pathological findings. The topics seem odd today: hysterical fever, the use of quinine in the treatment of pneumonia, experiments with sphygmography on the brain, fatty degeneration of the newborn, and modern female invalidism. However, she was read widely and was broadly critical of the science of medicine in her day, writing and speaking to serious concerns of the profession. Charles Loomis Dana, M.D., in his introductory note to the 1925 volume, *Mary Putnam Jacobi: A Pathfinder in Medicine,* wrote,

Dr. Jacobi added many clinical and pathological and educational facts which still remain valuable to her chosen science. She will be remembered by these and also by the example of her courageous and path-breaking career and by her success in promoting the elevation of woman's status as contributors to science and as efficient members of a learned profession.[20]

Her writings, as does her career, point to the admirable results to be expected from demanding the best from ourselves in our daily work as well as in our life with others.

3. The role of women. In those years of reform and growing demands for equality for women in both the public and private sectors, Putnam Jacobi and Elizabeth Blackwell provide polarized examples of responses to changing times. Two decades apart in age, they were colleagues at the Infirmary and respected each other highly. Putnam Jacobi, noting the importance of Blackwell, wrote that, "Among all the pioneer group of women physicians, hers chiefly deserves to be called the Record of an Heroic Life."[21] Blackwell, wary - perhaps even fearful - of feelings of sexuality according to her early diary, stressed the special attributes of women for sympathy and compassion for the

poor. She defined women's role as teachers of hygiene and healthful living to the urban poor and the new waves of immigrants; she stressed the part that women should play as specialists in women's diseases, and urged them to use their femininity to further their careers.

Putnam Jacobi, on the other hand, sought equality with men in her profession and also in her companionship with men on a personal level. In a letter to her mother from Paris at the age of 24, she wrote,

> I have no particular desire to marry at any time; nevertheless, if at home, I should come across a physician, intelligent, refined, more enthusiastic for his science than me, but who would like me, and for whom I should entertain about the same feeling I have for Haven [her brother], I think I would marry such a person if he asked me, and would leave me full liberty to exercise my profession.[22]

She was fortunate in her marriage to Abraham Jacobi. They had a passionate, if occasionally tempestuous, relationship which produced two children and an admirable couple.

A fascinating example of starkly different approaches to the management of a case is afforded in the medical account of Charlotte Perkins Gilman, an outstanding feminist writer who, in 1885, had a 'nervous breakdown' following the birth of a child. She was treated by S. Weir Mitchell, a prominent Philadelphia neurologist, an acclaimed novelist, and a close friend of William Osler. Mitchell was well-known for his "Rest Cure" for neurasthenia. His treatment consisted of enforced bed rest under the care of a nurse. Personal contact with family members was restricted, and crying was prohibited. This treatment was a clear development of Mitchell's severe Victorian feelings about the role of women based upon their physical oddities. Gilman, on the other hand, was a feminist strongly opposed to traditional Victorian valuation of gender roles. Her treatment by Mitchell failed miserably, and she sought out Putnam Jacobi in 1902. We do not know what her treatment method was, but we can infer the personal aspects that led to its success. Gilman wrote,

> When I met her I found we were more or less interested in the same things. She became most kindly interested in my variety of neurasthenia and made a proposition to me. She said she had originated a system of treatment which she desired to try for that ailment, and nobody would allow her to do so. I said I was perfectly willing to let her try it on me, and we formed a compact. She proceeded to develop with me the original system, and the result was admirable. I worked under her for some months, going to her office every day, and she put me through a course of most remarkable performances and gave me this compliment - that I was the most *patient*

patient she ever had. I found her the most patient physician I had ever known, and the most perceptive. She seemed to enter the mind of the sufferer and know what was going on there, and I have carried with me, and always shall, the deepest...feelings for that broad mind....Dr. Jacobi seemed to me an example of a free and original mind, thinking for itself and working out its methods, not only taking accepted knowledge on a subject, but adding to it.[23]

It would be difficult to find a more impressive commendation. Gilman took her experience and wrote a famous short story, "The Yellow Wallpaper," a beautifully written and impassioned account of her dismal experiences with the "Rest Cure" of S. Weir Mitchell.

All eras have their own problems, the solutions to which will surely differ in details based upon the idiosyncrasies of the moment. However, the personal characteristics of those called upon to resolve the complex and persistent dilemmas and distresses of the human condition are probably quite similar at their foundation. Certainly, Mary Putnam Jacobi exhibited many of these characteristics. She was a strong advocate for working girls and women, was a participant in the Working Women's Society and was vice-president of the Consumers' League for many years. Her colleague in this work, Florence Kelley, spoke of Putnam Jacobi's contribution:

She was a pioneer among physicians in going among working women not merely to cure, but to help *them* to change industrial conditions which create the need for cure, to help *them* make conditions of work such that disease and death need not be forced upon them.[24]

Putnam Jacobi was an ardent searcher for truth in terms of scientific facts, open to discoveries in physiology, pathology, and bacteriology that would revolutionize the practice of medicine. She was ceaseless in her encouragement of other women to become physicians on their own merits, and to enter the competitive professional scene confident in their education and training. She seemed to have had a sympathetic ear for patients as well as for students, family, and friends. Her life and her career are suitable models for students of any age and era.

In 1879 William Hurrell Mallock published a book, *Is Life Worth Living?* A staunch Roman Catholic, he decried the loss of public morality and personal behavior that seemed so prevalent in those years of confusing and frightening changes. He hoped for a return to a stronger Christian foundation for mankind. Putnam Jacobi responded to his essay with one of her own, a reply she titled, *The Value of Life.* In the concluding chapter she wrote,

The prize of life, or the object of living for each living being, consists in the development of all faculties to their greatest extent which the individual organization admits of, and in the satisfaction of all desires to their utmost possible capacity. The reason for failure and discontent will always be found in the fact, not that a "supernatural" stamp has been effaced, like a spurious watermark, from things which have been valued, but in the fact that some of these valued things have not been obtained, or that an imperfect analysis of the needs of human nature has caused the necessity for certain provisions for attainment to be overlooked.[25]

Jacobi closed her essay with these hopeful words for the Era of Reform:

And we may dare to say, that if society to-day be really in the position of a man who awakes from a dream, it is certain that any temporary regrets he may feel, must ultimately be more than compensated by the full possession of the dawning realities.[26]

---

[1]Putnam, Ruth, *Life and Letters of Mary Putnam Jacobi,* New York, G.P. Putnam's Sons, 1925, v-vi.

[2]Putnam-Jacobi, Dr. Mary, *From Massachusetts to Turkey,* League for Political Education Publication No. 1, 1896, 21.

[3]Jacobi, Mary Putnam, "Woman in Medicine," in *Woman's Work in America,* ed. by Meyer, Annie Nathan, New York, Henry Holt and Company, 1891, 144.

[4]Ibid., 144.

[5]Clarke, Edward H., *Sex in Education: A Fair Chance for the Girls,* Boston, James R. Osgood and Company, 1873, 17-18.

[6]Ibid., 39-40.

[7]Ibid., 127.

[8]More, Ellen S., *Restoring the Balance,* Cambridge, Harvard University Press, 1999, 8.

[9]Osler, William, in *In Memory of Mary Putnam Jacobi,* Academy of Medicine New York, New York, The Knickerbocker Press, 1907, 4-5.

[10]Jacobi, Mary Putnam, *The Question of Rest for Women During Menstruation,* New York, G.P. Putnam's Sons, 1877, 227.

[11]Ibid., 232.

[12]Jacobi, "Woman in Medicine," *op. cit.,* 198.

[13]Morantz-Sanchez, Regina Markell, *Sympathy and Science,* New York, Oxford University Press, 1985, 168-169.

[14]Ibid., 191-192.

[15]Jacobi, Mary Putnam, "Inaugural Address at the opening of the Woman's Medical College of the New York Infirmary, October 1, 1880," *Mary Putnam*

Jacobi: Pathfinder in Medicine, edited by the Women's Medical Association of New York City, New York, G.P. Putnam' Sons, 1925, 346-348.
[16]Jacobi, Mary Putnam, "Shall Women Practice Medicine?", *Pathfinder..., op. cit.,* 390.
[17]Jacobi, Mary Putnam, "Some Considerations on the Moral, and on the Non-Asylum Treatment of Insanity," *The Prevention of Insanity and the Early and Proper Treatment of the Insane,* Boston, Tolman & White, 1882, 12.
[18]Morantz-Sanchez, *op. cit.,* 194.
[19]Jacobi, Mary Putnam, *Physiological Notes on Primary Education and the Study of Language,* New York, G.P. Putnam's Sons, 1889, 120.
[20]Dana, Charles Loomis, "Mary Putnam Jacobi," in *Mary Putnam Jacobi: Pathfinder in Medicine, op. cit.,* xxxii.
[21]Jacobi, "Woman in Medicine," in Meyer, *Woman's Work in America, op. cit.,* 150.
[22]Putnam, Mary, in *Life and Letters of Mary Putnam Jacobi, op. cit.,* 141.
[23]Morantz-Sanchez, *op. cit.,* 213-214.
[24]Kelley, Florence, in *In Memory of Mary Putnam Jacobi, op. cit.,* 30.
[25]Jacobi, Mary Putnam, *The Value of Life: a Reply to Mr. Mallock's Essay, "Is Life Worth Living?",* New York, G.P. Putnam's Sons, 1879, 229.
[26]Ibid., 252.

Chapter 11

William James, 1842-1910

William James never practiced medicine. He graduated from Harvard Medical School in 1869 after a rather desultory career as a student. He then taught physiology and anatomy at the medical school for a few years at the request of the new president of the college, Charles William Eliot. Eliot had been professor of chemistry at the Lawrence Scientific School where James was a student in the early 1860s. This new school was established with a bequest from the textile magnate, Abbott Lawrence in 1847. Like the Sheffield School at Yale opened the year before, it had no formal ties to the college, but was begun as a response to the new and widespread interest in, and fascination with, science. A precursor of these schools, created in response to the same interests in science, was the Lowell Institute, a lecture series established in Boston in 1839 with funds from the will of another textile magnate, John Lowell, Jr. The Massachusetts Institute of Technology would be created by the state some two decades later.

As I have discussed before, revolutionary changes in the structures and the convictions of society are often unexpected occurrences at a time of security and comfort in current beliefs. The middle third of the nineteenth century was just such a remarkable period in America, a time of sharply polarized events. The ferocity of the Civil War, the literature of Lowell, Hawthorne, and Melville, the Transcendentalism of Emerson, Thoreau, Channing, Fuller and Alcott, the drive for abolition of slavery by Garrison and Parker, and the phenomenal growth of industrial power played off against each other as the nation began to receive the waves of massive immigration from Europe. For many Americans these years of the nineteenth century were an Age of Certainty, a time when the assurances of religious faith in a created and orderly world would be affirmed by the new discoveries of science that would provide comfortable confirmation of the significance and meaning of that physical world. The mutual supports provided by scientific knowledge and religious truth would establish the foundation for a just, reliable, and reasoned national society.

Both of these convictions would be shaken and then demolished as the century progressed. This unexpected loss of certainty was central to the developing thought of William James and a lesson for the education, training, and practices of physicians. The life and work of James present a model for physicians. He is a model, not because of his few years as an instructor in a medical school, but because of characteristics of his personality important for all professional persons. James held - in imaginative tension - his education, his ability to think, and his interpretations of actual experiences. He was able to create - not only himself as a new person - but also several impressive intellectual accomplishments: a school of philosophical thought influential in his time: Pragmatism; a textbook of psychology that offered new interpretations of our thoughts and acts; and a study of religious experiences still read today. William James moved on from an instructor in physiology to teach psychology, and then philosophy, at Harvard. He became a revered author and lecturer, and an internationally recognized, even adulated, figure of his time.

The Person

James was born in New York City, the eldest of five children. His next younger brother, Henry Jr., would become a leading novelist of his time, an author whose works are still widely read today, some translated into popular movies. Their father, heir to a large fortune, spent most of his life at home writing and supervising the education of his children. Captive to a powerful desire to separate himself from an inherited severe Calvinist Prebyterianism, Henry Sr. devoted his life to writing and lecturing in a tendentious manner about the need for freedom of the spiritual life from the prison of dogmatic religions. Henry Sr. was subject to fits of depression and panic attacks, a father who presented a seriously conflicted and confusing personality to his children. In 1844, while on a trip to Europe, he experienced a startling panic attack that he interpreted as a warning that his proud sense of knowing the 'truth' about faith was, in fact, a false sense of his importance and his interpretive skills. He found the writings of Emanuel Swedenborg and realized that he had suffered what Swedenborg called a "vastation." Henry Sr. became a devoted reader and exponent of the philosophy of this eighteenth century Swedish scientist and writer on spiritual experience. His son, William, would have a similar experience later.

Linda Simon, on the faculty at Skidmore College, described Henry Sr. in her 1996 book, *Remembering James.*

He preached tolerance but could be remarkably insensitive to the feelings of others; he wrote that human beings were essentially good, but felt that self-love would interfere with one's belief in the goodness of God; he wrote that children should be free to discover their own identities but exerted overwhelming control within his own family....He was, in short, a difficult man to have as a father, and he caused his children considerable distress. Even before the children could understand the ideas their father professed, they knew he had the power to interpret reality and manipulate their lives.[1]

The reader receives the distinct impression of a passive-aggressive personality destructive to those dependent on him. He smothered his children with what seemed affection; he was so possessive of *their* affection that he could not tolerate their attachment to teachers who were models. The children went from school to school, here and throughout Europe, never able to finish any program. Whenever they settled into a school and seemed happy and admiring of teachers, they would be moved to another school, often in another country. Their father's apparent lack of a career and his persistent demand that his children be free to do whatever they wished (as long as it was fully acceptable to him) sent a confusing and highly ambivalent message leading to William James' difficulties in deciding what to do with his life. One positive result was, however, that William learned the major European languages, an accomplishment that served him well in later years. The children responded to their father's control in varied ways: Henry moved to England; two sons, one a lifelong alcoholic, fought in the Civil War; a daughter who never married, had repeated psychotic episodes and died of breast cancer. She had submitted to implied parental desires and stayed home. William's career would be a remarkable journey.

William James' mother, Mary Walsh, provided the nurture and the stability for her children. Always supportive of her husband's odd ideas, she ran a 'tight ship' for the family, submitting to the strong paternalistic wishes of her husband while caring for their children. Their memories of her were positive and thankful.

William James suffered from panic attacks and depression - 'melancholia' - throughout his first thirty years. He had difficulty choosing a career: drawn to science *and* to philosophy, his father would, however, not permit him to go to Union College with a close friend to study engineering. Henry Sr. had graduated from Union after a profligate student life, and was concerned that William would succumb to the same temptations. His hopes for William lay in the study of science; he hoped that his eldest son would discover and present the certainties of scientific investigation that would prove the truth of the spiritual ideas that were presented by his new idol, Emanuel Swedenborg. Eugene Taylor, in his 1990 essay on the origin of William James's psychology in *Reflections on "The Principles of Psychology,"* wrote that

> Henry James Sr. and his transcendentalist friends advocated a spiritual evolution of consciousness that James the Elder hoped would be systematically elucidated in a set of definable laws by the new methods of scientific empiricism....Because the natural law was in fact derived from the spiritual, and not the other way around, he untiringly delivered his piquant barbs and thrusts to all who would demean this one great spiritual truth.[2]

His hopes for his son's uncovering of the scientific truth of his spiritual convictions would not be realized.

The Age of Uncertainty

Before discussing the education that William James received, I will set the stage for the intellectual revolution that was just underway when he started his studies at the Lawrence Scientific School in 1861. As I discussed previously, in the early decades of the nineteenth century many Americans went to Europe, particularly to Paris, Vienna, and Germany to study the emerging new laboratory sciences. They returned home enthusiastic about the potentials for understanding our physical world, healing the sick, and, for some, perhaps even providing a foundation for religious belief. In New England, in particular in Boston and Cambridge, there was a firm foundation in Puritanism and the new denomination, Unitarianism, religious orders that were open and hopeful that the new sciences would confirm with certainty the role of God in creating and sustaining the universe.

A cataclysmic event in this time was the publication of *Origin of Species* in 1859. Charles Darwin's book- the result of three decades of collection of specimens, study, and thought - shattered two seemingly fundamental beliefs common to most persons: 1), belief in a God who created the world as we see and know it today, confirming the biblical interpretation of reality, and 2), confidence that scientific experiment also revealed the same truths about the physical world. Darwin, with his phenomenal study supported by his collections and data, introduced the concept of *probability* as central to our knowledge of our world. Indeed, theory was the only way to construct any concept of reality.

There was no certainty. Paul Jerome Croce, in his 1995 study, *Science and Religion in the Era of William James*, wrote,

[T]he practice of science up to the 1860s had been veering away from fact gathering and proof and turning toward hypothetical constructions based on plausibility rather than certainty - trends that Darwinism underscored, exploited, and furthered....[T]he new theory of species development through natural selection shocked supporters and antagonists alike not only for its frankly naturalistic assumptions and bluntly antisentimental morality but also for its implicitly probabilistic methodology.[3]

In academic settings such as Harvard, *Origin of Species* provided a new way to study and interpret both science and religion. One could *believe* in God and in scientific truth, but neither was certain in human experiences. Coming from the laboratory or from theological studies, one could describe what was present in test tube or in human encounters with the Bible, but there were no explanations, only probabilities.

A Journey in Education

The early education of William James was sporadic and irregular. He studied at home and in a number of academies and schools as the family traveled to and from Europe. By his late teens he declared his interest in becoming an artist and studied at Newport under William Morris Hunt, an accomplished and popular painter. Henry Sr. was an advocate of Art in the abstract, but saw the artist as an artisan, a career unfit for his son. He took the family to Geneva, but finally returned to Newport in 1860 and William resumed his artistic studies with John La Farge as a fellow student. William became disenchanted with his future possibilities as an artist and, following up on his father's suggestion, enrolled as a student at the Lawrence Scientific School in 1861. Here he studied chemistry under Charles William Eliot who noted that James' skills were more in the area of observation than experimentation, that his earlier education had been spotty, and that James seemed to suffer from a nervous constitution. James spent two semesters there, took a semester off to be at home, and then returned to Lawrence, finally transferring to an anatomy course taught by Jeffries Wyman. Part of his reason for this transfer was having heard public lectures by Louis Agassiz, the renowned naturalist and director of the Museum of Comparative Zoology. Agassiz had strong religious convictions and believed that all species of animals and plants had been created by God as they appear now. His ideas received wide acceptance in the religious community of Boston. His theories and beliefs ran absolutely counter to the new theory proposed by Darwin, the concept of natural selection as a probable explanation for the origins of the species we know. James found himself located at the very center of the major scientific controversy of the century.

James was unsure of what career he should choose. He vacillated between becoming a naturalist studying under Agassiz, returning to art, becoming a doctor, or just doing nothing, living off his parents. Finally, without much enthusiasm, he chose medicine and began his studies in February 1864. The following year he took some time off and joined Agassiz on a trip to South America, an expedition that convinced him to abandon a career in the natural sciences. James' course through medical school was chaotic, interrupted by trips to Europe to treat his malaise and depression. In 1866 he did a summer internship at the Massachusetts General Hospital; in 1867 he was studying, half-heartedly, physiology in Germany. Finally, in 1869 he received his M.D. degree from Harvard.

During these student years of 1861 to 1869 James was friends with proponents of both sides of the arguments generated by Darwin's work. Agassiz, rejecting natural selection, was opposed by Asa Gray, an outstanding botanist at Harvard, and a confidant of Darwin. Gray was a prolific writer, accurate in his science and compelling in his arguments. An early opponent of Darwin was Oliver Wendell Holmes, professor of anatomy and physiology at Harvard. Suspicious of the growing interest in science, and an avid proponent of bedside teaching as the major channel for instruction, Holmes' views were reported by James in a 1868 letter to his parents. James noted that, in his *Introductory Lecture* to the students Holmes said, "the amount of baggage which a doctor is now expected to carry is growing too great....[I]t must be granted that by far the greater part of the matter recorded in physiological treatises has as yet found no application....We must not expect too much from 'science' as distinguished from common experience."[4] The student of today can only stare in disbelief at this assertion.

Among James' close friends were Charles Sanders Pierce, Chauncey Wright, and Charles William Eliot, all men who challenged each other with their knowledge and their reason. They would form the Cambridge Metaphysical Club in the 1870s, a forum for ongoing argument and definition of the meanings of the new sciences and the metaphysics from Europe. Another important teacher for James was Charles Edouard Brown-Sequard, Harvard's first professor of neurology, an experimentalist in the tradition of Claude Bernard. Bernard was one of the outstanding scientists in France who, by his experimental work, established physiology as an independent science. James was impressed by the methods and the thinking of both of these men, using their techniques of reasoning as the foundation for what would be his developed philosophy in the years to come.

After receiving his M.D. degree James was undecided on his future. He did not want to practice medicine, but did not know what else to do. Living at home, he became depressed. Writing to his friend and former fellow student, Henry Pickering Bowditch who was studying physiology in Germany, James suggested that they become partners: James would do the reading and Bowditch would care for the patients. This would not be acceptable to Bowditch, a nephew of Henry Ingersoll Bowditch, and a man who would become a leader in the field of physiology. In a later letter, James revealed his deepening depression when he suggested that Bowditch become superintendent of an insane asylum, and he, James, a patient.

In 1870 James probably reached the depths of his depression. Rand B. Evans, in his 1990 essay, "William James and His *Principles,*" wrote that "The illness was accompanied by a devastating fear of his own inability to control his own destiny." Evans continued with James' comment on reading an essay by the French philosopher, Charles Renouvier. James wrote,

> I think that yesterday was a crisis in my life. I finished the first part of Renouvier's second "Essais" and see no reason why his definition of Free Will - "the sustaining of a thought because I choose to when I might have other thoughts" - need be the definition of an illusion....My first act of free will shall be to believe in free will....[5]

The Career

In 1869 Charles William Eliot was appointed President of Harvard, introducing an era of renewed vigor in teaching, in science, and in faculty development. James, apparently looking back to his student days under Eliot, was not impressed; he found Eliot to be lacking in some of the gentlemanly virtues of tact and polite behavior. However, the appointment proved to be of benefit for James. When Bowditch was a student at Lawrence Scientific School Eliot had been impressed with his skills. When Bowditch completed his studies in Germany in 1871 he returned to Harvard, at the age of thirty-one, to be an assistant professor of physiology and the developer of projected new laboratory facilities. This would be a challenge since laboratories were essentially non-existent. Linda Simon, in her 1998 study of James, *Genuine Reality: A Life of William James,* wrote,

> Bowditch resumed his warm friendship with James. During the 1871-72 academic year, Bowditch welcomed James into his laboratory and his home, sharing with James his responses to recent works on physiology. As much as he respected James's sharp intelligence, he, like other accomplished friends, no doubt were mystified by James's inability or unwillingness to pursue a career. It seems likely that Bowditch was trying to give James's life some positive direction when, in the summer of 1872, Bowditch asked James if he would take a vacant course on anatomy....Eliot, who remembered James as a student, voiced no objection, and in August, James was offered his first professional job.[6]

This was the start of an illustrious career that began in anatomy and physiology and reached its fulfillment in psychology with the publication, in 1890, of *Principles of Psychology.*

James's course in 1872-73 in physiology was a success that cheered him and encouraged him to pursue an academic career. He went abroad again in 1874, and returned in 1875 to teach a course in physiological psychology for graduate students at the Lawrence Scientific School. This course firmly established his popularity as a teacher and he began his ascent of the professional ladder. He was appointed assistant professor of physiology in 1876, and the following year offered his course in psychology in the department of philosophy over the strong objections of the chair of the department, but with the support of President Eliot. Rand Evans offered this summary of James's progress:

> By the fall of 1879 James was teaching "Physiological Psychology" to graduate students, a course on Renouvier to seniors and a class on Spencer's *First Principles* to juniors....By 1889, James's title changed again, this time to professor of psychology. By then, James's version of the new psychology was firmly established at Harvard. His teaching and the articles that would come from his pen during the 1880s would establish him as one of the leaders of American psychology.[7]

James was instrumental in assisting the move of psychology from philosophy and religion to become a scientific and a clinical discipline. James, in his persistent search for his inner self and in his struggle to assert his free will to define his own life, finally achieved prominence and satisfaction as a teacher.

James was a prolific writer and a lecturer who hypnotized his students. A significant part of his teaching technique recalled by students was to request them to critique his lectures by writing comments and making suggestions for improvement. He was a relaxed instructor, informally dressed, freely open to discussion and argument. Not only with students, but with colleagues and other writers, dialogue became a core part of his teaching and writing careers. He also became a well-known and idolized public speaker, addressing audiences across America and in major European cities. He popularized philosophy and psychology at a time - the Progressive Era - when confidence in bettering the self was as common as the conviction that America would continue to prosper.

James delivered the prestigious Gifford Lectures on Natural Religion in Edinburgh in 1901 and 1902, one of the highlights of his career. He struggled for two years in their writing, spending a year in Europe undergoing spa treatments for a cardiac condition suggestive of angina pectoris. The writing of these lectures was important to James. Linda Simon noted that

> The Gifford lectures were his chance - perhaps, he thought, his final chance - to reconcile for himself the questions of faith that always had been central to his philosophy. As he mined autobiographies, confessions, popular self-help books, and serious studies of theology, he sought to understand how "a broken and contrite heart," such as his own, could achieve solace through some manner of faith, through some "transempirical" experience. A sense of yearning underlay James's writing: in nearly thirty years, he had not overcome the feeling...of being "separated from God."[8]

These lectures were published as James's most popular book, widely read to this day, *The Varieties of Religious Experience.* He remained well-known and respected as a teacher, retiring from Harvard in 1907. His health declined rapidly and he died of cardiac failure in 1910. In the last few years of his life his reputation fell off; his attempts to write a final and definitive treatise on his philosophy of Pragmatism were unsuccessful.

Lessons from His Life and Work

Although James did not pursue a career in medicine, his life and his thought have much to teach physicians. An outstanding literary critic and teacher, Alfred Kazin, in an essay in his 1997 book, *God and the American Writer,* commented,

What James did, very much in the American style, was to *appeal* his life, to open it up with the same candor and directness with which he opened up all his thought in its many successive stages in order to *save* it, literally, by the power of his thought. As experience in all its possible departments and ramifications became the foundation of his teaching as a philosopher, so personal experience became the underlying strength of his work. One reason why he became famous as much for his temperment as for his philosophy is that he pursued his thought...for readers and listeners who perhaps recognized his problems as their own. The most important thing to recognize in this reliance on particular ideas for dealing with oneself as a creature always in crisis - James's particular importance to us - is that it candidly looks on religion as therapy.[9]

One of James's lessons for us is the need to understand the self, to be alert to the nuances of our interior life as they reflect - and reflect upon - our professional life. Although James was uncertain about the sharp focus Freud placed upon sexuality as determinant of our psychological development, he was convinced of the certainty of the subconscious self, italicizing the phrase in his writing. This 'inner self' was an ongoing concern for James and Mark Twain who were good friends, having met in Florence in 1892 while on vacation. They were both interested in psychic research and were members of the Society for Psychical Research. They knew each other's writings, and frequently shared their concerns about religion and the inner life. In a 1996 study, *Mark Twain and William James,* Jason Gary Horn related their 'experienced selves.'

As with Twain, private experience lies at the heart of James's theory of religion, in which religion functions as a part of this inner experience rather than as a force acting upon it from without. For James, religion is intensely personal and functions both as a mediator of experience and as experience itself. As James said in his *Psychology,* religion provides the means of coalescing the self with the divine across an ever-shifting felt fringe of psychic relations.[10]

James placed religion in the realm of therapeutic method. He was concerned with the function of religion as a way of understanding the self, of using the temper of religious thought as a contemporary way of finding another avenue to the unconscious self, a way to further development and maturation of that self in a confusing world in which final knowledge is withheld. His *The Varieties of Religious Experience* remains popular because James described and discussed the psychological problems and conundrums with which religions are concerned.

In the Age of Uncertainty in which James lived and worked, science was the source for concerns about the values of the personal self, the individual life. Bruce W. Wilshire, in his Introduction to the 1984 book, *William James: The Essential Writings,* described the problem.

> James was convinced that science had generated a nightmare of alienation for man. In the ordinary nightmare we have motives but no powers; in the scientific nightmare we have powers but no motives....[W]e wander detached, our emotions merely subjective....How can life be significant and activity worth the bother if human dreams and emotions are nothing but by-products of systems that are describable, predictable, and controllable without any reference to them at all?[11]

Another point in James's psychology-philosophy is his setting aside the dry theories of personality and of logical thought. Instead, he stressed the role of experience in determining who we will become as persons. If we are to continue learning and developing professional skills we must constantly evaluate our experiences to ensure that theory and experience confirm - and not contradict - each other. James's philosophy - Pragmatism - was an effort to reject closed systems of thought by making the longing for a true knowledge of reality a possibility. Linda Simon described the hope of this philosophy:

> For James, pragmatism tempered empiricism with humanism; the observer, the thinker, the seeker after truth, was necessarily implicated in the process of inquiry and experimentation. Pragmatism, then, invested each individual with the authority to determine truths; privileged what James called "percepts" over abstract concepts; and linked philosophical decisions to moral actions.[12]

A significant part of that evaluation is understanding the roles of our personal reactions to those experiences in determining our interpretations. Continuing study is essential. James was convinced that life is deeper and more meaningful than is generally recognized; it is essential to our development to be steadily analyzing our experiences and our responses to them if we will become more capable in our work, more sensitive in our relationships, and more convinced of our ability to serve and to love.

James found life to be filled with mystery; not only the incongruities of human behavior, but the natural world as a steady source of amazement. The human body is astounding; the human mind and the psyche are equally undecipherable, yet so determinative of who we are and will become. James was an early observer of what we call 'stream of consciousness' thought. "Consciousness," he wrote, does not appear to itself chopped up in bits. Such words as 'chain' or 'train' do not describe it fitly as it presents itself in the first instance. It is joined; it flows. A 'river' or a 'stream' are the metaphors by which it is most naturally described. *In talking of it hereafter, let us call it the stream of thought, of consciousness, or of subjective life.[13]*

We live in an era in which science and technology are definitive of our understanding of our selves and our world. We rely on science to determine our daily existence in almost all areas: medicine, agriculture, transportation, education, entertainment, and the provision of our everyday needs. James, with his introduction to science through the study and teaching of anatomy and physiology was aware of, and appreciated, science. He did, however, question what is commonly called, the "objectivity" of scientists. This question continues to our day. We are uneasy accepting the claim of strict disengagement of scientists from their work and from the significance of that work for us. The philosopher should be conscious of, and alert to, the self in all its relations. Bruce Wilshire, in his Introduction noted above, wrote,

> James would remind us that philosophy requires remarkable individuals willing at some points to take risks in achieving closure in their thought and in locating their existence;...A philosopher is a lover of wisdom, his subject matter is ourselves - and at closest range, and with relentless claim upon him, his own self....He must try to tell us where we are, who we are, and what we are to do....Philosophy involves engagement, leap and choice; it is intrinsically dramatic.[14]

I do not think it is a great leap of the imagination to define the good physician in similar terms of perception of self and of others, of engagement in the lives and experiences of others, and in commitment to the good of those in care. At the conclusion of his Introduction, Wilshire noted that "Perception for James is art-like, and perception as involving action figures in the ground of that developmental continuity which is the good life."[15]

James - based I am sure upon his years of growing up with his neurotic father - was acutely conscious of his experiences in his life. Periods of severe depression for many years, contemplated suicide, and marked confusion about a role for him in society that would be valid - all these exerted powerful influences on his developing thought and purpose. He referred, again and again, to 'experience' in laying out the tenets of his thought. In his writings he stressed the need to accept individual interpretations as accurate and real readings of that individual. All judgments of other persons are, not only questionable, but hazardous. Our knowledge must be constantly questioned and revalued as both new knowledge and new experience correct it. James saw the person as a totality: an amazing, quixotic, and often confusing reality. The life and the thought of William James remain important teachers for us. Although many of his ideas are idiosyncratic and related to his time, there is a foundation there for us. Alfred North Whitehead, a leader in philosophic thought in his time, delivered a series of lectures at Wellesley College in the 1937-38 academic year. In his first lecture he said,

> In Western Literature there are four great thinkers, whose services to civilized thought rest largely upon their achievements in philosophical assemblage;...These men are Plato, Aristotle, Leibniz, and William James.[16]

Whitehead continued by describing the contributions of William James:

> [T]he essence of his greatness was his marvelous sensitivity to the ideas of the present. He knew the world in which he lived, by travel, by personal relations with its leading men, by the variety of his own studies....His intellectual life was one protest against the dismissal of experience in the interest of system.[17]

It will be difficult to find a more reasoned description for the life hopes and expectations of the dedicated physician.

---

[1]Simon, Linda, "Introduction," *William James Remembered,* Lincoln, Nebraska, University of Nebraska Press, 1996, x.
[2]Taylor, Eugene, "New Light on the Origin of William James's Experimental Psychology," in *Reflections on "The Principles of Psychology,"* edited by Michael G. Johnson and Tracy B. Henley, Hillsdale, NJ, Lawrence Erlbaum Associates, 1990, 34.
[3]Croce, Paul Jerome, *Science and Religion in the Era of William James,* volume I, Chapel Hill, The University of North Carolina Press, 1995, 227.
[4]Ibid., 146.
[5]Evans, Rand B., "William James and His *Principles,"* in *Reflections on "The Principles of Psychology,"* op. cit., 21-22.
[6]Simon, Linda, *Genuine Reality: A Life of William James,* New York, Harcourt Brace & Company, 1998, 132.
[7]Evans, *op. cit.,* 24.
[8]Simon, *Genuine Reality, op. cit.,* 296-297.

[9]Kazin, Alfred, "William James: Rescuing Religion," *God and the American Writer,* New York, Alfred A. Knopf, 1997, 163.

[10]Horn, Jason Gary, *Mark Twain and William James: Crafting a Free Self,* Columbia MO, University of Missouri Press, 1996, 16.

[11]Wilshire, Bruce W., "Introduction," *William James: The Essential Writings,* Albany, State University of New York Press, 1984, xxi.

[12]Simon, *Genuine Reality, op. cit.,* 346.

[13]James, William, "The Stream of Thought," *The Principles of Psychology,* in *William James: The Essential Writings, op.* cit., 53.

[14]Wilshire, "Introduction," *op. cit.,* lxi.

[15]Ibid., lxiv.

[16]Whitehead, Alfred North, *Modes of Thought,* New York, The Macmillan Company, 1938, 3.

[17]Ibid., 4.

Chapter 12

Richard Clarke Cabot, 1869-1939

Richard C. Cabot was born in Brookline, Massachusetts, the fifth son of seven in a prominent Boston Brahmin family. His father was a philosopher, a friend and biographer of Ralph Waldo Emerson, and an Overseer of Harvard College. His mother, Elizabeth Dwight, was a devout Christian. Together these parents provided a secure and comfortable environment for their sons. The intellectual and religious climate of their patrician home provided the setting in which a moral sense of duty was instilled in their son, Richard, whose interests in religion and philosophy led to a degree in philosophy, *summa cum laude,* from Harvard College in 1889. In his early college years Cabot planned on becoming either a Unitarian minister or a professor of philosophy. In the summer before his senior year, however, he met Dr. E. L. Trudeau, the sanatorium physician, at the family's Adirondack summer house near Saranac, New York. In conversation with Trudeau, Cabot realized that the life of a physician offered ample opportunity for a very practical way to help people in need. Cabot changed his professional goal and graduated from Harvard Medical School in 1892.

Cabot was an innovative thinker alert to what was happening in his time and place. A new member of a profession not renowned for envisioning changes in social, economic, and medical methods and goals, Cabot matured and did his major productive work in the Progressive Era of 1890 to 1920. These were years of enormous migration: there was a steady movement of rural families to the cities in search of work; there was also the arrival of some 17 million persons from Europe in two decades, mostly to industrial cities. This astounding movement produced a profound layering of the population. Ida M. Cannon, a nurse who would become a social worker at the Massachusetts General Hospital (MGH) in 1907, and subsequently head of the social service department for thirty-one years, described her experience that moved her toward social work. She was a visiting nurse in the river slums of St. Paul, Minnesota. As a student in sociology at the University of Minnesota she heard Jane Addams speak of the hazards of life in the slums and the factories. Moved by

Addams' quiet passion, Cannon began a new journey. She observed in her 1952 book, *On the Social Frontier of Medicine,* that

> Jane Addams awakened in me, as she did in many, a realization of the gross inconsistencies in our so-called democracy. It was obvious that there existed side by side, desperate poverty and vast wealth, illiteracy and our acclaimed system of free public education, abundant production for our use from industries that maintained hazards for those who worked in them: all these existed in our land while we in self-satisfaction assumed that "all's right with the world."[1]

This, then, was the world Cabot entered as he completed medical school. He did an internship for eighteen months at the MGH and then spent a year as a fellow in hematology research. He published his first paper, "Leukocytosis as an Element in the Prognosis of Pneumonia." Although he went on to do some further work and published an early textbook of blood disorders four years later, his experiences confirmed his commitment to patient care, and he began his medical practice. As a response to his learning experiences in the laboratory, Cabot remained critical of any effort to separate laboratory 'facts' from clinical 'facts' in their importance for the care of patients. In a 1904 article in the *Boston Medical and Surgical Journal* he spoke to the "harm done by the attempt to separate our examination of the patient's functions into two sharply differentiated portions and to assign one portion to the individual known as the laboratory man, and the other portion to someone called a "clinician,"....[2] Cabot would try to hold these areas in balance in his work in both the clinical and academic spheres. He was appointed to the position of Physician to Outpatients in 1898, beginning his long association with the hospital and the medical school.

His appointment occurred at the time in medicine when advances in the sciences made new methods of diagnosis and treatment possible. Cabot observed that

> these new resources have also complicated the work of the physician in a dispensary, and made it more difficult for him to remember each patient and all the details about each patient as the physical, chemical, psychological, biological facts emerge in the complex ramifications of modern diagnosis and treatment.[3]

Medical practice in the city also was changing. The new emphasis on the importance of science was apparent in the type of office practice that became common. Laboratory studies of blood and urine were introduced into offices, improving the diagnostic capabilities of doctors. It was a time when, thanks to the new ease of traveling from town to town, patients began to shop for doctors. "As the century closed," physician-historian Christopher W. Crenner suggested in his 1993 doctoral thesis at Harvard,

> a greater range of people began to shop for the doctor's services. A variety of people were traveling into the city to find proper care and following their leads whenever they needed to.
> A new word emerged...for this new behavior. Patients called what they did "doctoring" and this usage rose to standard recognition during the heyday of Cabot's private practice....
> Doctoring by 1900 meant to visit doctors, but it also carried an ironic warning about the difficulty facing women in their encounters with Victorian medicine....Doctoring did not cure what ails you....Doctoring was used particularly when one subjected oneself to available treatments in vain[4].

Cabot was an advocate of group practice, the assembling of physicians with various specialties and varied interests to offer patients the best available resources for both diagnosis and therapy. He noted that the poor and the rich had access to the best of care, the former in university dispensaries, the latter from multiple consultations. It was the people of 'moderate means' who suffered from lack of competent services. Cabot was not speaking of group practice of the private office type, but used the Mayo Clinic as his example of the possibilities opening up for better options for the middle classes. He noted the hostility of private practitioners to the competition, but pointed out the obvious advantages to the patient of

> a group who work together as a team, each doing the part that he has fitted himself especially to do and dove-tailing in with the work of others similarly skilled in other fields...especially now when the complications of medical diagnosis and the varied types of skill needed in medical and surgical treatment are becoming more and more elaborate.[5]

Very early in his career Cabot was sensitive to the many factors that influence diseases in causation, in treatment, in coping, and in caring for the seriously ill. In addition to his office practice, Cabot's entire medical life was spent at the MGH. His early work at the turn of the century in the Outpatient Department was a watershed event, introducing him in a profound way to the powerful influences of social, psychological, and financial factors on the health of his clinic patients.

Awakenings

Reflecting on those early days, Cabot recalled his futility in his work, his sheer inability to attend to the needs of the hundreds of patients who came to the clinic daily. The importance of his reflections on his sense of inadequacy points to his growing awareness of all those other aspects of personhood that influence health and illness. It was apparent to him that he knew nothing about his patients' families, living conditions, work situations, income, or nutrition.

> Treatment in more than half of the cases that I studied involved an understanding of the patient's economic situation and economic means, but still more his mentality, his character, his previous industrial history, all that had brought him to his present condition, in which sickness, fear, worry, and poverty were found inextricably mingled....[6]

Cabot found his frustrations to be intolerable: unsure of his diagnoses, treatments seemed haphazard; superficial knowledge of his patients made him doubt his accuracy. Even treatments that were prescribed might very well not be carried out. The events of the day were working in his favor, though. Where previously the Dispensary was a place where drugs that matched the presenting symptoms of the patient were 'dispensed,' the new association of outpatient facilities with university medical schools brought trained and competent physicians whose hopes and expectations were for providing comprehensive care.

Reflecting on his personal and professional experiences led Cabot to think about ways to eliminate the frustrations that so annoyed him and to make these important personal factors of medical care available to the other physicians working in the OPD. The developing and self-defining profession of social worker would provide an answer.

Social Work

The middle years of the nineteenth century were a time of contentious debate and argument in efforts to understand the care of the poor. England was the center of these early attempts to define who was entitled to free care. In 1869 the London Charity Organization Society was formed to organize existing relief agencies and work toward improving the living conditions of the wretched masses in the world's greatest city. An important - and distressing - aspect of these efforts was the resistance of physicians to the provision of free care for the poor; they were concerned that their incomes would be reduced! However, there were physicians who understood the questions that plagued Cabot in Boston: poverty, work, family, social supports. A Medical Committee of the London Society was created with the purpose of defining methods of determining who was entitled to care, with or without fees. Over the next twenty years a plan was developed and implemented, and as a result of the labors of Charles Loch by 1895 there was an almoner [one who distributes alms to the poor] working at the Royal Free Hospital. Her duties were to screen patients for their ability to pay and, as important, to refer families to relief agencies for assistance. Within the next decade seven other London hospitals had appointed almoners, and the position of Hospital Almoner was firmly in place.

In the United States a similar effort was begun at the New York Infirmary for Women and Children by Elizabeth Blackwell. Home visitation by the women physicians was encouraged and, in 1866, a Sanitary Visitor was appointed, Dr. Rebecca Cole, the first black women to become a physician in the United States. Her duties were to study and document the home conditions of their patients and teach hygiene, nutrition, and other essentials for good family health. The New England Hospital for Women and Children under the supervision of Dr. Marie Zakrzewska soon followed suit, encouraging home visits by both doctors and students. In Baltimore, with the combined efforts of the new medical school at Johns Hopkins, the YMCA, the Emmanuel Church and the Charity Organization Society, medical students visited tuberculosis patients at home to teach proper care and assist them in finding support for living. In 1908, the first social worker was appointed at the Johns Hopkins Hospital.

In several American cities that had settlement houses - Boston, Chicago and New York - workers learned of the social conditions of the poor by living in close proximity with them. But, as Ida M. Cannon pointed out,

> more special training obviously was needed for those who would deal constructively as well as sympathetically with individuals in distress. In the summer of 1898, the New York Society had offered a six-week session for students of "philanthropy." This summer school continued yearly until 1904 when, through an endowment, the New York School of Philanthropy (later called School of Social Work) was established.[7]

Richard Cabot was a director of the Boston Children's Aid Society. In his characteristic way he volunteered to work with some of the boys so that he would learn about the functions of the Society. In those days, as pointed out above, social workers were employed by charitable organizations to study the needs of the community. Cabot learned, as he listened to the 'case presentations,' that social workers collected and analyzed the very information that he lacked in his clinic work. Bringing the skills and abilities of social workers into the hospital setting became a possibility for him. To provide a statistical base for his contention that social needs were as important as physical diseases in bringing persons to the OPD, he did an analysis of the patients he saw during a year's work there. In his paper, "Suggestions for the Reorganization of Hospital Out-Patient Departments, 1906," he wrote,

> To find the cause of disease, and remove it when possible, is the first principle of all rational therapeutics....When malnutrition is due to poor appetite and poor sleep, and when these, in turn, appear to result from worry, our pledge to be thorough, to go to the bottom of the patient's malady, find its cause and root it out, compels us to undertake through others (nurses or social workers) investigations for which we dispensary physicians have neither time nor training.[8]

Cabot found that, of some 4300 patients he had seen in 1904, 59% had physical diseases, and 41% had what he labeled, 'functional' diseases. In this latter category were diagnoses such as constipation, debility, neurasthenia, alcoholism, headache and other pains without known cause, dyspepsia, and cardiac neurosis. These findings, in addition to the work he did with the Children's Aid Society, convinced him of the need for social workers in the Dispensary.

This was a watershed time for social workers as they clarified their role in relation to the role of psychiatry, a profession undergoing radical reorientation itself. Medical historian Elizabeth Lunbeck, in her Introduction to her 1994 book, *The Psychiatric Persuasion,* observed that

> In the early years of the twentieth century...American psychiatry was fundamentally transformed from a discipline concerned primarily with insanity to one equally concerned with normality,....[T]hey laid new conceptual foundations for their specialty, delineating a realm of everyday concerns - sex, marriage, womanhood and manhood; work, ambition, worldly failure; habits, desires, inclinations - as properly psychiatric and bringing them within their purview.[9]

The evolving profession of social worker was strongly influenced by this change of label from alienist - therapist to the insane - to psychiatrist - therapist of the neurotic normal person. One of the major influences of psychiatry, according to Lunbeck, was to help "the psychiatric social worker...to suppress the censorious judgments of the dissolute and feckless that her disciplinary forebear, the friendly visitor, had reflexively issued."[10]   Social work and practice were fundamentally changed thereby, opening up a new approach to caring for persons seeking help from physicians at dispensaries and hospitals. The sharp focus of the doctor on the physical symptoms of the patient can deflect attention to other personal needs that psychologically trained personnel can see and help. In their 1936 book, *The Art of Ministering to the Sick,* Cabot and a Protestant minister, Russell L. Dicks, pointed out some of these needs.

> We work hard to improve the condition of the sick man's body, but we allow conditions to exist which hurt his mind and through his mind check the healing of his tissues....We ignore the patient's view of hospital sights, sounds, and smells, of the doctor's significant silences and half-heard conversations....[11]

In 1905 Cabot brought, under his own auspices, Garnet Isabel Pelton, a nurse who was a resident of a settlement house and knowledgeable of social issues, to the clinic at MGH, gave her a desk in the hall, and she began to work with the physicians. The following year he hired Ida M. Cannon who had come to study at the Boston School of Social Work and would work for MGH for nearly forty years, most of the time as chief of the Social Service Department, formalized in 1921.   The introduction of social work to the hospital, both in-patient and out-patient, was a major contribution of Cabot to health care reform in the twentieth century. In his presidential address to the Eighth Congress of American Physicians and Surgeons in 1910, E. L. Trudeau commended Cabot.

> It is to this high type of optimism that we owe, through the untiring labors of Richard Cabot, the social service department of the tuberculosis dispensary. The success of Dr. Cabot's work has been due primarily to his own personality, which so strongly reflects his faith and his ideals, and which inspires those efforts he directs. This new departure in medical work is not scientific in character, but Christian and humanitarian. It is being taken up as a regular part of every modern dispensary and hospital, and extended to relief measures among children, chronic invalids, and convalescents, and promises in time to revolutionize the whole character of hospital and dispensary methods.[12]

The advent of Christian Scientists in Boston, various cults such as Mind Curists and other "irregulars" recalled the earlier nineteenth century threat of alternative therapists that I presented in previous chapters.   John Harley Warner, in his 1986 study, *The Therapeutic Perspective,* noted the decline in power and status of the professions in America in those years.

> In medicine...regular physicians believed that their profession as a whole had been debased in the public view. Populistic medical sects such as Thomsonianism, as well as sects like homeopathy that appealed to a more affluent clientele, challenged both the orthodox profession's claim to intellectual and therapeutic superiority and its economic well-being.[13]

Most physicians deplored these sectarian options, but Cabot saw them as confirmation of his observations about inadequate medical care that did not take account of the social and psychological aspects of human nature.   Cabot's own personal religious convictions and experiences increased his awareness of these parts of ourselves.   In 1909 he noted that

> Every candid physician knows that fear causes some disorders, that self-absorption causes others, that sin and half-smothered remorse cause still others. But he is afraid to admit the full consequences of these truths....He calls it rubbish or sentimentality or superstition or simple ignorance....
>   The enormous influence of spiritual environment, of friendship, of happiness,   of   beauty,   of   success,   of   religion,   is   grievously underestimated....There   are   diseases   that   cannot   be   cured   without friendship, patients that never will get well unless you can get them to make a success of something or to conquer their own self-absorption by a self-devotion, losing their life to find it.[14]

The Career

Cabot, as I noted, had done laboratory work and published his results while a Dalton Fellow, shortly after finishing his internship. He was well aware of ongoing advances in physiology, pathology, surgery, and bacteriology and in his writings supported the growing use of the new laboratory sciences for diagnosis and for screening in medical care, both in his practice and his clinic work. He was, however, cautious about the new-fangled notions of Sigmund Freud who gave his American lecture debut in Worcester in 1909, but Cabot was certainly alert to what he called "'psychical" influences on the health of his patients.

One of the grand inheritances from the middle years of nineteenth century medicine was the concept of *vis medicatrix naturae* - the healing power of nature. Jacob Bigelow, in his 1835 lecture on the nature of disease, focused sharply on this concept, and it achieved more and more acceptance over the next decades. Cabot was a firm believer. In the book referred to above co-authored with a Presbyterian minister-chaplain, Cabot recalled

> I went into medicine in the hope of helping people. I found that I could help vastly less than I hoped. I was not wise enough to help as I wanted to. But though I could give a great deal less, there was a great deal more for me to receive. There was more for me to learn and to be inspired by as I watched the behavior of this extraordinary creation we call the human body....[15]

Cabot recalled that his student years, his internship, and his subsequent medical practice in clinic and in office provided sufficient examples of the power of nature to heal disease.

In a chapter, "The Two Must Face a Third," in their book just referred to, Cabot wrote about a potentially catastrophic and not uncommon current problem in modern psychotherapy: "The disaster most to be feared by the minister who visits the sick is that patients, especially women, will fall in love with him." He continued with the question, "How are we to give our best service over months to sick women without creating an emotional dependence not to be distinguished from falling in love?" He discussed various methods to prevent intimacy with patients, fully recognizing that "sex tends to make two persons strongly aware of each other and oblivious of the rest.[16] One third person to be recognized could be to recall the spouse not present; another third person present in the relationship between patient and physician is God, a healing presence Cabot believed to be central to many of the 'cures' doctors achieve.

The Teacher

A major part of the professional life of Cabot was spent in teaching. He stressed the importance of instruction for all professions involved in medical care, particularly in times of rapid advances in the physical sciences, in psychology and psychiatry, and in the social sciences, all of which have an impact on patient care. In one of his later books, the 1931 volume, *Social Service and the Art of Healing,* Cabot was quite explicit, again speaking to issues of abuse and neglect current to our times.

The truth is, that before proper and helpful co-operation of doctor and social worker can be established each of the two must educate the other considerably - perhaps painfully. The social worker must be led to understand, for example, how often "laziness" is a sign of disease rather than of sin and how devious and unexpected are the paths by which sex-tension connects itself with cruelty, with "nervousness," and with slipshod habits. The doctor must be helped to see how a patient's physical good may have to be sacrificed temporarily in order that a job may not be lost or a family broken up.[17]

An important tool for teaching in medicine and the other professions is called the Case Method. Developed at the Harvard Law School, it was picked up in 1900 by Cabot and one of his students, Walter B. Cannon, later to become a distinguished Harvard physiologist. The Case Method presented students with descriptions of actual medical and surgical cases, providing clinical descriptions from physical examinations and laboratory findings. Students then discussed these cases, offered diagnostic possibilities and treatment options, awaiting the final word from the instructor. Cabot's first collection of these cases, *Case Teaching in Medicine,* was assembled in 1906, and published in 1908. Cabot appreciated the fact that medical knowledge could be gathered from books and from lectures. His central concern, however, was how to get medical students to *think.* In his Introduction to the textbook Cabot pointed to its purpose.

> After the student has learned to open his eyes and see, he must learn to shut them and think, and when he is thinking the less he has to distract him the better.
> To aid the teacher in training his pupils to think clearly, cogently, and sensibly about the data gathered by physical examination is the object of this book.[18]

There were a number of subsequent editions of this textbook, and the popularity of the method spread rapidly to other schools.

In 1910 the Case Method was expanded into one of the major teaching devices in modern medicine, the very famous and effective Clinical-Pathological Conference or CPC. This powerful teaching method was started by Cabot after a patient treated as a neurasthenic was found to have died of cancer. The CPC went one step further than the Case Method in teaching: in the conference a case, usually a complicated and confusing one, was presented and discussed by clinicians. Laboratory and X-ray findings were given and, finally, the pathologist discussed the findings at biopsy or autopsy. The CPC was a process whereby students at all levels of training and practice could learn from a careful study of documented materials, and have the opportunity to match their diagnoses against the findings of the pathologist. This teaching device continues to this day, published in each issue of *The New England Journal of Medicine* as "Weekly Clinicopathological Exercises FOUNDED BY RICHARD C. CABOT."

The role of the physician as teacher was important in Cabot's professional experiences. He wrote,

We all have a latent desire to teach somebody something. No physician lacks the opportunity....His patients always look to him for instruction; indeed, they almost force it out of him....

This part of medical work grows more and more important every day, for preventive medicine, the livest of modern hopes, is built up not only through public instruction, but especially through the lessons passed on individually by doctors to their patients and through them to families and neighborhoods.[19]

Cabot advanced steadily in his work at MGH. In 1912 he became Physician and Chief of the West Medical Services of the MGH, and in 1918 was advanced to Clinical Professor of Medicine at Harvard Medical School. In that same year he wrote a lengthy essay, *Training and Rewards of the Physician*. In this essay he detailed most of the components of what he considered the good physician's personal, as well as professional, life. He advised his readers on proper conduct, the 'tricks of the trade' of practice, the foibles of doctor and patient, and many other aspects of the daily routine of medical work. Cabot was concerned, not only with how to be a good doctor, but also with our human traits and characteristics that will cause failure. He wrote,

Many men fail because they do not keep up with medical progress. Every young man thinks when he graduates and settles down to practice that he is going to devote a good deal of time to reading. But as the years go on, he devotes less and less until today probably the medical reading of the majority of physicians in this country consists in skimming very hurriedly the titles or contents of one medical journal a week.[20]

This advice remains most appropriate for persons in all professions today, and probably indefinitely. The revised medical curricula for medical schools that followed upon the Flexner Report of 1910 were influenced by the writings of Cabot as they were by the groundbreaking work of William Welch and William Osler at Johns Hopkins. Another important recommendation of Cabot was the importance for the young physician of joining the staff of a hospital where contacts with colleagues would encourage learning of new advances in both medical science and practice.

The Person

In a remarkable address, *Truth and Falsehood in Medicine,* given as one of the Cartwright Lectures at the Academy of Medicine in New York in 1902, Cabot took a strong stand against the use of placebos, and for the telling of the truth to patients. This was quite remarkable in his time when it was considered compassionate care to withhold bad news from patients. Cabot's experiences over many years led him to the conclusion that lying was never justified. Obviously, there are different ways to tell the truth to others, and he discussed them. He concluded his talk by stating

> I will sum up the results of my experiments with truth and falsehood, by saying that I have not yet found any case in which a lie does not do more harm than good....The technic of truth telling is sometimes difficult, perhaps more difficult than the technic of lying, but its results make it worth acquiring.[21]

In 1919 Cabot left the MGH to become professor of social ethics at Harvard, allowing him to devote his remaining academic years to ongoing studies of the moral, religious, and philosophical bases for medical practice and the relationships among patients, associates, and community. His persistent interests in these areas were developed by him in a discursive and rambling textbook, *The Meaning of Right and Wrong,* published in 1933, six years before his death. At the end of the book he presented his concept of what he called, supermoral, that human characteristic of heroism, of doing more than would ordinarily be expected of us. He wrote, "What is it that such a man desires when he commits himself to the mercy of fortune for the love of a mere abstraction: justice, truth, life? He desires to do and to endure whatever this abstraction demands."[22] There is a delightful late Victorian flavor to this writing; it is also, however, a sincere and a defining characteristic of the personal and the professional life of this man.

As always, any study of the past can inform the present and warn the student at any level of learning that much of what is taken for truth and reality today is, in fact, only partly true, perhaps even incorrect. Any student of history is brought up short over and over again by reading of the obvious and undebatable 'truths' of medicine in our history:

theories of diseases and therapies that are ludicrous today were unquestioned in the not-too-distant past.

Cabot was an outstanding man of his time and of his professions. He showed our propensity for 'knowing' more than is known. Opinion becomes fact, and the urge to teach and to profess hypotheses as truths is given in to over and over again. Cabot showed us the interior strengths needed to learn and to heal, to witness and to support, to struggle and to be a hero. His writings also show us our common fallibilities and our assumptions of truth that turn out to be error.

In 1919 Cabot delivered the Ether Day Address at the MGH. Recognizing the high standards for behavior and for study of the institution, Cabot listed them:

> [T]he wise man's honest confession of ignorance, the absence of suspicion, secrecy and backbiting, the rule of fairness to others, the habitual thoroughness of examination, record and subsequent study, the habitual courtesy under conditions which tempt us to a bald and mechanical type of intercourse,....[23]

Cabot, perennially observant of himself and his companions in medical practice and teaching, commented on the ongoing need for combining persistent study and service to assure steady growth as a physician and as a person: "I have found in all the deeds by which men live, one salient feature, - the responsive interplay between purpose and fulfillment, between initiative and return."[24] To me, Cabot was a man who lived out a life that mirrored Henry David Thoreau's hopes for his own. In reviewing his 'experiment' at Walden Pond, Thoreau advised his reader "that if one advances confidently in the direction of his dreams, and endeavors to live the life which he has imagined, he will meet with a success unexpected in common hours."[25]

---

[1]Cannon, Ida M., *On the Social Frontier of Medicine,* Cambridge, Harvard University Press, 1952, 39-40.

[2]Cabot, Richard C., "The Ideal of Accuracy in Clinical Work: Its Importance, Its Limitations," *Boston Medical and Surgical Journal,* CLI:21, November 17, 1904, 560.

[3]Cabot, Richard C., *Social Work: Essays on the Meeting Ground of Doctor and Social Worker,* Boston, Houghton Mifflin Company, 1919, xii.

[4]Crenner, Christopher W., *Professional Measurement: Quantifying Health and Disease in American Medical Practice,* Ph.D. Thesis, Harvard University, Cambridge, Massachusetts, 1993, 142, 146.

[5]Cabot, R. C., *Training and Rewards of the Physician,* Philadelphia, J. B. Lippincott Company, 1918, 124.

[6]Cabot, Richard C., *Social Work: Essays on the Meeting Ground of Doctor and Social Worker, op. cit.*, xxiv.

[7]Cannon, *op. cit.*, 45.

[8]Cabot, Richard C., *Suggestions for the Reorganization of Hospital Out-Patient Departments, 1906,* in *Richard Cabot on Practice, Training and the Doctor-Patient Relationship,* edited by John Stoeckle and Lawrence A. May, distributed by Dabor Science Publications, Oceanside, NY, 1977, 114-15.

[9]Lunbeck, Elizabeth, *The Psychiatric Persuasion,* Princeton, Princeton University Press, 1994, 3.

[10]Ibid., 160.

[11]Cabot, Richard C., and Dicks, Russell L., *The Art of Ministering to the Sick,* New York, The Macmillan Company, 1936, 6.

[12]Trudeau, E. L., *The Value of Optimism in Medicine,* The President's address at the Eighth Congress of American Physicians and Surgeons in Washington, May 2, 1910, Saranac Lake, 10.

[13]Warner, John H., *The Therapeutic Perspective,* Princeton, Princeton University Press, 1997, 38.

[14]Cabot, Richard C., *Social Service and the Art of Healing,* New York, Dodd, Mead & Company, 1931, 23-24.

[15]Cabot and Dicks, *op. cit.*, 118.

[16]Ibid., 172, 175.

[17]Cabot, Richard C., *Social Service and the Art of Healing, op. cit.,* 183-184.

[18]Cabot, Richard C., *Case Teaching in Medicine,* Boston, D. C. Heath & Co., 1908, vii.

[19]Cabot, *Training and Rewards..., op. cit.,* 146.

[20]Ibid., 70.

[21]Cabot, Richard C., *The Use of Truth and Falsehood in Medicine: An Experimental Study,* in *Richard Cabot on Practice, Training and the Doctor-Patient Relationship, op. cit.,* 262-263.

[22]Cabot, Richard C., *The Meaning of Right and Wrong,* New York, The Macmillan Company, 1933, 435.

[23]Cabot, Richard C., *The Achievements, Standards and Prospects of the Massachusetts General Hospital,* Ether Day Address, October 16, 1919, 7.

[24]Cabot, Richard C., *What Men Live By,* Boston and New York, Houghton Mifflin Company, 1914, 330.

[25]Thoreau, Henry David, *Walden,* edited by J. Lyndon Shanley, Princeton, Princeton University Press, 1989, 323.

Chapter 13

Alice Hamilton, 1869-1970

At the beginning of the Introduction to her 1984 book, *Alice Hamilton: A Life in Letters,* historian Barbara Sicherman wrote,

> No one did more during the first half of the twentieth century to alert Americans to the danger of industrial diseases than Alice Hamilton. A physician and reformer, she specialized in industrial toxicology, a branch of public health that investigates the hazards to workers of poisonous substances used in manufacturing. If she did not single-handedly found the field, as has sometimes been claimed, she was its foremost practitioner in the early years of this century.[1]

The life of Alice Hamilton is instructive for us in its depiction of a woman born and raised in the Victorian Era who became an acclaimed physician in a specialty she helped define. She was apparently without fear in her repeated confrontations with the impressive political and financial powers of the day, and she incorporated her experiences - medical, social, political, and personal - into an admirable model for any person dedicated to the application of knowledge and compassion to the improvement of the health and the general welfare of others.

Hamilton was born and raised in Fort Wayne, Indiana. She had three sisters: the eldest was Edith, a scholar and headmistress of the Bryn Mawr School in Baltimore and the renowned author of books such as *The Greek Way* and *Mythology.* None of the four daughters married, a situation that, in our time, might raise questions about the behavior and role of a strict Presbyterian father unsuccessful in business and a heavy drinker. There was a fifth child, a son, born when Hamilton was seventeen, a quiet and polite man. Hamilton, in keeping with many in her generation, thought that women were more sympathetic and wiser than men and struggled with the question of how far women should go to follow men in career choices and in social behavior. The end of the nineteenth century was a time when the roles of women were sharply debated: to seek a profession or care for one's parents; to choose work or marriage; to emulate the male role model or seek fulfillment in creating a new female role as yet undefined?

Hamilton attended Miss Porter's School in Farmington, Connecticut, as did ten women - sisters and cousins - in her family. While her sister Edith chose teaching, Alice chose medicine for her career. She described her reasoning for her choice:

> I chose it because as a doctor I could go anywhere I pleased - to far-off lands or to city slums - and be quite sure that I could be of use anywhere. I should meet all sorts and conditions of men, I should not be tied down to a school...or have to work under a superior....[2]

Hamilton returned to Fort Wayne, studied the sciences she had ignored at Miss Porter's and entered the medical department of the University of Michigan at Ann Arbor in 1892. Two of her teachers in this outstanding school, John Abel and William Howell, would shortly afterwards join the faculty at the new medical school at Johns Hopkins. Hamilton did well, chose the scientific laboratory side of medicine rather than the clinical, and graduated in 1895. She and Edith went to Europe for a year where, as women, they struggled for acceptance as students. The German universities at Munich and Leipzig were strongly resistant to admitting women to either lectures or laboratories; women could not attend autopsies. Alice accomplished little in the laboratories where she worked. She returned, spent a year at Hopkins working with the pathologist Simon Flexner, and published a paper on tubercular ulcers in the stomach. In 1897 she accepted a position in pathology at the Woman's Medical School at Northwestern University and moved to Chicago.

Hull-House

In 1889 Jane Addams and Ellen Gates Starr opened Hull-House, a 'settlement' on the west side of Chicago. They purchased an old mansion that would become the center of community life for the poor. Madeleine P. Grant recounted the establishment of Hull-House in her 1967 biography of Hamilton.

> After months of careful searching they came upon a red-brick mansion built by Mr. Charles J. Hull in 1846. It had been his suburban home, and he had hoped to attract other wealthy men to build in the same area. Instead, the rapidly growing industries of Chicago had moved in and swamped it. In one direction were the stockyards, in another the shipbuilding yards on a branch of the Chicago River. Between these, there was a six-mile slum area where thousands of immigrants lived and worked.[3]

Hull-House, and hundreds of settlement houses like it in the many tenement sections of American cities, also became home for educated young persons eager to serve the poor and to experience the adventures of the ongoing drives for reform.

As I have noted, the years 1830-1850 in America were characterized as the initial years of an era of reform. There were many movements dedicated to change - to an uplifting - in both the spiritual and the secular segments of society. The causes supported ranged widely: women's rights, temperance, universal education, prison reform and the abolition of capital punishment, improvement of the conditions of the working classes, and, of course, the abolition of slavery. There were no mass followings for these causes, and, in America, there was a distinct religious character to them. After the Civil War these reform movements accelerated, and public health concerns, especially for the working poor, became critical.

It was to these reform efforts that young women and men responded and sought out institutions such as Hull-House. Some of these volunteer workers stayed for a few years, others for decades. Alice Hamilton came to live there in 1897, and did so for more than twenty years while she developed the new profession of industrial medicine physician. Hull-House provided adult education, baths, well-child care, meeting facilities for social reform programs, a gymnasium, kindergarten, classes in subjects ranging from mechanical drawing to Dante and Greek art, and many other community services that the city ignored. Central to its purposes was serving the poor as advocates of a better life for them. Hull-House would become the most famous American settlement house. When Hamilton moved in there were twenty-five residents who, working at a variety of jobs in the city, volunteered their services of teaching, organizing, canvassing, lecturing, and representing the poor in their struggles for work and food. In the heart of a tenement section, poverty, tuberculosis, high childhood mortality, and despair were daily reminders for the residents of their purposes in their work with the poor.

Hamilton had serious doubts about her abilities and her goals. She had difficulty integrating the scientific aspect of her work in pathology with the service component at Hull-House, finding neither one self-defining in itself, yet both important for her fulfillment as a person. The sterility of laboratory work bored her. But the self-sacrificing part of settlement work pointed up a role expected for women that she was determined to avoid. Her question was, for those years, how to combine service and science into her life in a way that would make that life worthwhile, both for her and others? Whatever thoughts she had about her decision to forego marriage and childrearing we will not know. She noted at one time that she was looking forward to getting old.

In 1902 Rush Medical School of the University of Chicago began admitting women; one consequence was that the Women's Medical School of Northwestern closed. Hamilton took a job as bacteriologist in the new Memorial Institute established by Mr. and Mrs. Harold McCormick to study scarlet fever, the disease that killed their son. In the fall of the year, an epidemic of typhoid fever occurred, with a high incidence of cases in the nineteenth ward, the location of Hull-House. Hamilton did a study of cases, and determined that improper sewage disposal was the cause, and that the disease was spread by flies. Quantities of captured flies confirmed the presence of the bacillus on them. She presented her finding before the Chicago Medical Society in January 1903, and her paper was published the next month in the *Journal of the American Medical Association.* A furor resulted with slanderous attacks on the study, but health reforms did occur with the appointment of a new Commissioner of Health. As it turned out, the real cause of the epidemic was a broken water main that permitted sewage to seep into the water supply of the ward. This event was Hamilton's introduction to public health matters, and over the next few years she studied cocaine use, and helped organize a committee on tuberculosis prevention for the Visiting Nurse Association. In 1907 she served on a committee sponsored by Hull-House and the Chicago Medical Society to improve the training of midwives. Wilma Ruth Slaight, in her 1974 doctoral thesis, *Alice Hamilton: First Lady of Industrial Medicine,* detailed some of the findings of the committee:

> [L]aws covering licensing of midwives absurdly inadequate and outdated. Many of the practicing midwives had little or no training; others were found lacking in cleanliness, some to the point of constituting a danger of infection to their patients. One-third were classified as criminal, either because they constituted a physical danger to their patients or because they, alone or in conjunction with a physician, defrauded their patients or participated in illegal abortions.[4]

These activities introduced Hamilton to reform circles and she began to write articles for the social work press on her findings, gaining recognition for her studies.

The Dangerous Trades

Hamilton became interested in industrial diseases through her residence at Hull-House. She wrote,

Living in a working-class quarter, coming in contact with laborers and their wives, I could not fail to hear tales of the dangers that workingmen faced, of cases of carbon-monoxide gassing in the great steel mills, of painters disabled by lead palsy, of pneumonia and rheumatism among men in the stockyards.[5]

She read a book, *Dangerous Trades*, by Sir Thomas Oliver, an Englishman instrumental in cleaning up the lead industry in Britain. This book sent her off to the library to read about dangers industrial workers encountered. She was amazed to find that all the literature was European. The silence in American medicine was deafening: no texts, no medical meetings, no physicians for whom this was a specialty except men employed by the industries. These "contract" doctors, as they were called, were usually looked down upon by other physicians as men incapable of enduring the demands of regular medical practice. This was probably in 1907.

Next came the reading, in 1908, of a manuscript by John Andrews, executive secretary of the American Association for Labor Legislation. He had investigated the use of white phosphorous in the match industry and documented 150 cases of what was called, "phossy jaw," the progressive destruction of jaw, face, eye, and occasional blood poisoning from exposure to phosphorus. Although known for fifty years, almost nothing had been written in American medical literature; European literature, by contrast, discussed treatment and methods of prevention. Following publication of Andrews' paper, legislation effectively made the use of white phosphorus untenable.

There were other stirrings about the hazards for the laborer, man or woman. The relationship between tuberculosis and occupation, the increased hazards for working women, and the dangers of the mines and steel works were topics of increasing concern among reformers. Interest in sickness insurance for the workers, in place in many European countries, sparked concerns here and, in 1908, the governor of Illinois appointed an Occupational Disease Commission, the first in the United States. This was encouraged by a friend of the governor, a sociology professor at the University of Chicago, Charles Henderson, also a friend of Hamilton. Thanks to that association, she was appointed to the Commission, and in 1910, became its medical investigator. Hamilton wrote,

We were staggered by the complexity of the problem we faced and we soon decided to limit our field almost entirely to the occupational poisons, for at least we knew what their action was,...Then we looked for an expert to guide and supervise the study, but none was to be found and so I was asked to do what I could as managing director of the study with the help of twenty young assistants, doctors, medical students and social workers.[6]

The Commission divided up its duties and Hamilton was assigned to study lead poisoning. The Commission members visited plants which they had to find on their own since the State Factory Inspector's office was of no help! Sicherman noted that Hamilton

> began by trying to determine which Illinois industries used lead. Starting with the known users, she picked up gossip about other likely sources....Hamilton and her assistants visited 304 establishments and discovered more than seventy industrial processes that exposed workers to lead poisoning.[7]

The young assistants scoured hospital records, talked with doctors, pharmacists, and labor leaders looking for cases. From case records Hamilton went to their homes and, through these interviews, learned about the uses of lead. Perhaps the finding that surprised her most came from a home visit to a patient who pointed out to her that the enamel finish on bathtubs was produced by sprinkling enamel dust - rich in red oxide of lead - on red-hot tubs. A sample of the dust contained 20% lead. This led Hamilton to the conviction that lead poisoning is caused by breathing in dust, and not failure to wash one's hands properly, the usual explanation offered by factory managers to explain the poisonous effects of lead. Lead is one of the oldest industrial poisons, known to the Romans and included by Pliny in the diseases of slaves who were potters and knife grinders. Hamilton's conclusion was that

> there can be no intelligent control of the lead danger in industry unless it is based on the principle of keeping the air clear of dust and fumes....A hundred years ago Tanquerel des Planches, who is called the Columbus of lead poisoning, noted that severe plumbism never followed the handling of solid lead but only exposure to dust and "emanations."[8]

The report of the Commission was presented to the governor in 1911, demonstrating clearly that there were thousands of cases of lead poisoning - even deaths - in the state. Within months Illinois passed an occupational disease law, one of only six states to do so. Sicherman noted,

Hamilton's study of white lead...conclusively demonstrated the prevalence of lead poisoning in the industry. Visiting all but three of the seventy-five known American white-lead factories, she documented 358 cases of poisoning, including sixteen deaths, that had occurred in a sixteen-month period. Even by this early date, she had developed the techniques that would become her trademark: thorough investigation of factories, correlation of illness with specific industrial processes, and compilation of medically diagnosed cases of lead poisoning.[9]

Hamilton presented a paper, "The White Lead Industry in the United States," at the Second International Congress on Occupational Accidents and Diseases in Brussels in 1910. There she met Charles P. Neill, the United States Commissioner of Labor, who, the following year, invited Hamilton to do a national study of the lead industries. Her study included the paint industry where lead was the major ingredient. One of her discoveries was the use of sanding between coats of paint. The Pullman car industry drew her attention: the painters stood in the cars sanding the interiors before the next coat of paint could be applied. The air was thick with the dust of lead paint. The automobile industry was a major interest also. Ford cars received fourteen coats, Packards nineteen, with sanding often done between coatings.

One of the alarming findings that Hamilton made in her lead industry studies was the insignificance of lead poisoning to the companies. On her visit to Salt Lake City, she wrote to her mother

I am amazed to see how lightly lead poisoning is taken here. One would almost think I was inquiring about mosquito bites....When I went through the records of the wards maintained in one of the hospitals by that smelting company, I realized why it seemed so unimportant, the accidents are so terrible and so numerous that a little thing like lead colic attracts no attention. My hair almost stood straight as I read of the burnings and crushings and lacerations, the amputation of both arms, the loss of eyes, the deaths from ruptured livers and intestines.[10]

Perhaps the most distressing finding in all of her early studies was the initial indifference of factory owners and managers to the multiple hazards of their industries. It is difficult for us today to comprehend the significance of a twelve-hour day and a seven-day week, particularly in work that involved very hard physical labor. Another factor that Hamilton realized was the disregard that owners and managers, as well as governments and police, had for immigrants. This is a very large sector in the revealing work of Hamilton. She wrote,

I used to despair of relief for the overworked, underpaid immigrant laborers, who took with hopeless submission whatever was given them, who rarely ever dreamed of protesting, much less rebelling. It was they who did the heavy, hot, dirty, and dangerous work of the country. In return for it they met little but contempt from more fortunate Americans....The Carnegie Company's principle of a high tariff to shut out cheap foreign-made goods, and a wide-open door to let in cheap foreign labor, resulted in the building up of great fortunes; but measured in terms of human welfare it was cruel and ruthless.[11]

Hamilton continued in her work in the years up to the end of the First World War. One of her assignments was to study a condition among stonecutters called, "dead fingers." The introduction of the air hammer, while greatly increasing the work output of the laborers, required holding the drill portion tightly in the hand, causing what Hamilton called "spastic anemia." This was a condition in which the tightness of the muscles in the hand shut off the flow of blood to the fingers. This did not seem to be the type of industrial hazard that Hamilton was accustomed to study. What Hamilton did note, however, was the high incidence of pulmonary disease among the men who cut granite and marble, including increased rates of tuberculosis. This confirmed her belief in the role of respiration in causing deadly illnesses. The air hammer, in another setting, was just as serious a concern. Copper miners in Arizona used the air hammer to break up the rock. Beginning with holding the hammer against their thighs, they often let it slip up to the abdomen and the chest wall with resultant strange sensations within their bodies that they interpreted as injury. Hamilton assured them that their bodies would not suffer from the air hammer. The dust produced by their work would prove to be the danger with which they lived.

The war years brought a new demand on American industries, the production of explosives. Most of the chemicals used in this industry came from Germany; with the blockade by the British, American manufacturers had to start up new factories without the experience of the Germans. The use of nitrates, of picric acid, and of mercury introduced a variety of poisons requiring new and untried methods of control, not only of the combustible materials, but also of the gases produced in making nitroglycerine and other explosives. The British had studied extensively the different forms of TNT poisoning and published their findings: liver failure and aplastic anemia were causes of death. Of this, American doctors knew nothing. Hamilton was distressed by her findings and wrote,

Our students unearthed some very shocking conditions, under criminally negligent doctors, all of which they reported to us, but even the committee backing me [The National Research Council] was not influential enough to bring about reforms....[I]t was impossible to overcome the arrogance of the manufacturers, the indifference of the military, and the contempt of the trade-unions for non-union labor.[12]

In her studies of the manufacture of explosives in 1915 Hamilton first observed the use of mercury fulminate as a booster to set off a bomb or shell. Later, in 1923, she was asked to investigate other uses of mercury in industry. Mercury, in its liquid molecular state, is called quicksilver and was mined in Spain as far back as Roman times. The ore - mercury sulphide - is harmless; quicksilver, on the other hand, becomes volatile at 40 degrees Fahrenheit, and is quickly absorbed both by the lungs and by contact with the skin. For miners, when "the silver runs free," that is, when there is quicksilver in the ore, they can be at risk. Mercury was used in the manufacture of lamp bulbs, batteries, thermometers, and, interestingly enough, the production of felt. The United States, after Spain and Italy, is the third largest source of mercury.

In the seventeenth century the Huguenots developed a secret formula, using a mercurial fluid, to make felt from animal fur. This process, using mercury nitrate, continued and was the method employed in Danbury, Connecticut, the 'fedora capital' of America. In the complex process of manufacture using heat and extensive hand labor, mercury is vaporized and absorbed by the workers. Symptoms, as might be expected with heavy metals, are mostly neurological with tremors and jerking of arms and legs, difficulty speaking, and most distressing, symptoms of mental instability with depression, overwhelming fears, excessive irritability, and a sense of unworthiness. This syndrome led to the well-known phrase, "mad as a hatter." Hamilton's interest and studies in mercury poisoning led to an invitation to become medical consultant to General Electric, a major manufacturer of lamps, a position she kept for ten years.

Personal and Social Issues

Alice Hamilton became the leading authority on lead poisoning in the United States and an accepted authority on industrial diseases by 1915. Commenting on profound changes in Hamilton, Sicherman wrote,

In her forties, she had finally discovered her true vocation. Her initial forays into the field had been marked by characteristic tentativeness and self-doubt. But it soon became apparent, even to her, that no one knew more than she did....To one who had always emphasized her own limitations, this hard-won confidence was profoundly liberating.[13]

Hamilton was able to witness with her life and her work to a commitment to help those who were unable to help themselves: immigrant laborers, women, and children - all persons who were ignored by the industrial giants of the time. The casual attitudes that employers took to their workers dismayed her, and strengthened her willingness and her ability to confront powerful men. Also, her exceptional skills provided entry into what was accepted as a thoroughly masculine world. Sicherman continued in her discussion of this aspect of Hamilton's life:

The work also permitted her to escape the constraints customarily imposed on women of her class without violating her own notion of femininity....[S]he delighted in her newfound ability to go anywhere and do anything a man could do;...Although she chose to work for the most part in a world of men, by emphasizing the human side of science and by relying on personal persuasion as an instrument of change, she was adopting a classically "feminine" strategy.[14]

In her approach to this demanding work that called into question many of the basic tenets of American industrialism and free enterprise, Hamilton's method of confrontation with potentially negative forces offers us a view of a technique for facing opposition: assuming a genderless approach to situations where argument and disagreement seem inevitable. For a physician, her approach seems impeccable. Sicherman observed that Hamilton's

greatest assets were her evident sincerity and her ability to meet the employer on his own ground. Convinced that any man of goodwill would do the right thing once he knew the truth, she had an uncanny ability to appeal to the best instincts of others. Her persistence and persuasiveness, combined with her carefully assembled evidence, helped to overcome the doubts and suspicions of many owners.[15]

Certainly this is sound advice for establishing a firm therapeutic relationship between physician and patient.

In 1915 Hamilton joined fifty other American women at an International Congress of Women at the Hague. This was the beginning of her lasting interests in peace and pacifism, international health, women's suffrage, and the complexities of post-war political issues. The actual support behind her involvement with these issues seems to have been Jane Addams, a phenomenally powerful person whose interior strength and commitments made her apparently without fear when confronting "the powers that be." They supported the League of Nations, and Hamilton was on the Health Committee of the League. One of the more important causes they supported resulted from the blockade imposed on Germany after the armistice of 1918. In their effort to force Germany to sign the Versailles Treaty, the Allies prevented any food from entering Germany, resulting in widespread starvation, especially of children. Addams and Hamilton joined forces with the English Quakers in an unsuccessful attempt to end the blockade. These acts, and many others, characterized the life of Hamilton, and suggest the developed internal strength that she learned could be counted upon.

The Harvard Years

David L. Edsall, Jackson Professor of Clinical Medicine at Harvard, knew Hamilton through their work on a National Research Council committee. He established an industrial disease clinic at the Massachusetts General Hospital and a degree program in industrial hygiene at the medical school. When he became dean of the medical school in 1918 he offered Hamilton an appointment as assistant professor in industrial medicine. She accepted the position, on a half-time basis, the next year; she was still committed to field work for the Department of Labor, for whom she was studying carbon monoxide poisoning and the hazards of the aniline dye industry. Hamilton was the first woman appointed to the faculty of Harvard University, a situation that proved uncomfortable in all social and academic environs due to the powerful ant feminine feelings of the all-male faculty. She survived, however, as might be expected from her previous encounters with hostile men in the industries she studied.

The next decade was a turbulent one. The labor union movement had been crushed by Carnegie and Frick in 1904, and later by Gary and Schwab in 1919. The twelve hour-seven day week would not end until the 1920s. A very strong isolationism developed in the United States that encouraged resentment and violent opposition to anything vaguely suggesting communism and resistance by the working class. Efforts to work with the League of Nations were opposed, and international concerns - both industrial hazards and social reforms - were set aside by powerful conservative forces.

Hamilton was associate editor of the *Journal of Industrial Hygiene* edited at Harvard, and was responsible for securing important articles for the journal. In a most remarkable reversal of industrial stance that displayed her abilities and stature, Hamilton was able to secure funding from several lead companies for a three-year study of the physiological and pathological effects of lead. Her first book, *Industrial Poisons in the United States*, was published in 1925. These years were ones of phenomenal growth in industry with a comparable growth in the number of toxic agents used. A new factor that increased the hazards for workers was the introduction of solvents that vaporized rapidly, placing poisonous agents into the air workers breathed. Through her years at Harvard - she retired in 1935 - she maintained very close contact with investigators and their legal attempts to improve the conditions of workers. Hamilton also continued her involvement with organizations such as the League of Women Voters, the Women's Trade Union League, and the Women's International League for Peace and Freedom. She never abandoned her concerns for international cooperation in these humane endeavors.

In the late 1920s investigation of the effects of radium on women employed in painting watch dials was begun. Workers used very small brushes which they dipped into radium, then used their lips to focus the brush before painting the numbers to make them luminous. The ingestion of radium led to its deposition in bone, providing a permanent source of irradiation to the body. Cancer and destruction of the jaw and face occurred, and many other conditions now known to be associated with exposure to radiation. The manufacturers blamed these on other circumstances. It would take several more years and legal action before this hazard would be acknowledged by the U. S. Radium Corporation in New Jersey. The historian Claudia Clark, in her 1997 study, *Radium Girls,* noted that

> Through remunerated scientific consultants, radium businesses were able to control knowledge about radium poisoning, concealing data that supported its existence and promoting opinions that put the blame for the dial painters' illnesses elsewhere.[16]

This example confirmed for Hamilton her observation when she wrote her book in the early 1940s that

> It is a pity that I cannot recall any instance of help from the organized industrialists to obtain for American workmen the sort of protection provided years ago in European industrial countries. But the truth is that the National Association of Manufacturers has fought the passage of

occupational disease compensation as it has fought laws against child labor, laws establishing a minimum wage for women and a maximum working day.[17]

Hamilton continued her work until her retirement from Harvard in 1935. Her second book, *Industrial Toxicology*, had been published in 1934. She was a recognized and influential woman in the field of industrial hygiene, lauded by both colleagues and by some of the major industrialists who realized her contributions to the safety and the welfare of all: manufacturers, workers, and also their families. Her last toxicology study was done in 1937-1938, an investigation into the effects of carbon disulfide, a chemical used originally in the vulcanization of rubber, but recently introduced in the manufacture of viscose rayon. Carbon disulfide causes a variety of mental disease conditions (delirium, tremors, mania) and was studied in Germany, France, and England in the middle years of the nineteenth century. Hamilton was successful in getting the industry to abandon its use after studies were done at the University of Pennsylvania Medical School. A recurring and distressing aspect of this saga is the reluctance of workers ill from the chemical to enter a study for fear of losing their jobs.

Hamilton visited Germany in 1933 and in 1938 and was horrified by the violence, the anti-Semitism, and the disintegration of a culture she had admired in the past. She was in Frankfurt for a meeting of the International Congress of Occupational Accidents and Diseases; Jews, Russians, and Czechs were absent, and Hamilton was the only woman present at the meeting which took place, amazingly, during "Munich week." Her experiences in Germany led her later to support American entry into World War II in fervent hope that a reconstructed Europe could result from victory. She retired, with her sisters, to their home in Hadlyme, CT on the Connecticut River.

Commentary

The story of Alice Hamilton engages the reader in a narrative that takes one back in time to an era - the Gilded Age - when rampant capitalism showed little regard for the men and women whose labors made its wealth possible. This sketch of her professional life shows a woman succeeding in finding a career that met her interior needs for accomplishment, and her hope to prove that women were the equals of men in her profession; gender differences are important in determining the self and our modes of interaction with others, but cannot restrict our choices of career or commitment. Hamilton had a deep desire to be of service to the needy of her time and she acted upon that desire.

There is almost nothing known of her private life: the customary roles for women of marriage and childrearing, voluntary service in the community, and instructors of the moral foundations of society. Her compassion for the immigrant laborer and the dispossessed of our nation, and her ability to stand up to some of the most powerful men of her time combine to offer us an example of the successes that can be known by adherence to conviction of purpose added to certainty of knowledge through experiment and experience. It might seem that she entered into her work at a special time and in a special place - the era of reform and at Hull-House under the tutelage of Jane Addams. These opportunities are available at all places and in all times. Her lesson for us might be that we are to see what is there before us, train ourselves to do the work that must be done, and then to persevere in its progress.

At the conclusion of her doctoral thesis, Wilma Slaight pointed out some of Hamilton's goals:

[S]he wanted to do more than merely secure the nation's physical well-being. She tried to improve the quality of life for its individual members. To this end she advocated birth control, worked for world and industrial peace, tried to insure fair treatment of immigrants from other lands, and worked consistently for the protection of the civil liberties of all. For Alice Hamilton individual worth and human dignity were not mere phrases.[18]

---

[1]Sicherman, Barbara, *Alice Hamilton: A Life in Letters,* Harvard University Press, Cambridge, Massachusetts, 1984, 1.
[2]Hamilton, Alice, *Exploring the Dangerous Trades,* Little, Brown and Company, Boston, 1943, 38.
[3]Grant, Madeleine P., *Alice Hamilton: Pioneer Doctor in Industrial Medicine,* New York, Abelard-Schuman, 1967, 56..
[4]Slaight, Wilma Ruth, *Alice Hamilton: First Lady of Industrial Medicine,* Ph.D. Thesis, Case Western Reserve University, 1974, University Microfilms, Ann Arbor, MI, 31.
[5]Hamilton, *op. cit.,* 114.
[6]Hamilton, Ibid., 119.
[7]Sicherman, *op. cit.,* 157.
[8]Hamilton, *op. cit.,* 122.
[9]Sicherman, *op. cit.,* 166.
[10]Hamilton, *op. cit.,* 151-152.
[11]Hamilton, Ibid., 6-7.

[12]Hamilton, Ibid., 197-198.
[13]Sicherman, *op. cit.,* 180.
[14]Sicherman, Ibid., 181.
[15]Sicherman, Ibid., 168-169.
[16]Clark, Claudia, *Radium Girls,* Chapel Hill, NC, The University of North Carolina Press, 1997, 2.
[17]Hamilton, *op. cit.,* 12.
[18]Slaight, *op. cit.,* 202-203.

Chapter 14

Postscript

This book is presented as a study of the renaissance in American medicine that occurred in the century between 1830 and 1920. What I have attempted to depict through analyses of the lives and the careers of these women and men is an era of renewed intellectual and professional activity that led to a new image of the physician in both the eyes of the public and the minds of doctors. This century was replete with ambivalent events. It is remembered as years that witnessed the Civil War and Transcendental literature and philosophy, the First World War and Existentialism, massive immigration and industrial expansion, exploitation of labor and reform in many areas, and - of central import for this study - the renewal of medicine. This vigorous renewal was the work of many physicians alert to the new advances in the sciences that forced reconsideration and revaluation of diagnostic and therapeutic methods currently in use as accepted and correct. The definition and the role of the medical school underwent complete revision as scientific discoveries encouraged the universities to develop medical departments and invest their resources, both financial and academic, in this renewed profession.

The word, renaissance, means a return, a rebirth, a revitalization of intellectual and artistic vigor. In medicine this does not imply a return to the ways by which medicine was practiced in some prior time. It does mean a return to high standards of education, and the application of the best of investigative skills to an understanding of the many and varied problems we face as persons and as communities. And, as always, this rebirth occurs as the result of the work of persons alert to winds of change that blow through our world. It is difficult to date changes since their precursors are seldom obvious and apparent to most of us. Thus, we study the past looking for clues to our present.

Permanence and Change

One of the important characteristics of history, and particularly the history of medicine, is the coexistence of stability and change. Just when we think we can relax and enjoy the constancy of the *status quo,* transmutations and alterations occur that startle us with their innovation and unimagined potential for further learning. It is the unexpectedness of the events that surprises us: especially in the general field of biology, but particularly in human physiology, where new findings require that we re-think fully accepted doctrines, concepts, and methods of practice.

The authority of our teachers plays a role in our resistance to new knowledge. And that authority, as we know in our history, goes back to the dawn of medicine. Galen and Hippocrates were fully acknowledged sources of the "biological sciences" and of medical treatment for countless generations of doctors. Whether it be parent, tribal priest, rabbi, judge, or professor of medicine, attention is paid to authority that appears to be based upon both knowledge and experience. One of the gifts of historical study is the power of learning to recognize the perennial fact of change.

In any profession, but particularly in medicine, keeping up with advances in the basic sciences is difficult. One of the problems is that what was known to be true yesterday is called into question today and is shown to be in error tomorrow. Particularly in the newer fields such as genetics, neurophysiology, and cell biology the reports of research are complex and often unintelligible to practicing physicians years out of medical school. In the nineteenth century, those early discoveries offered very limited therapeutic possibilities; there were almost no possibilities for medical interventions based upon them. It was a common opinion among physicians to find them interesting, but of no empirical value. In fact, one of the hallmarks of the educated and trained doctor at the turn of the century was what was called, 'therapeutic nihilism,' a pervasive sense of the lack of value of most therapies. In the twenty-first century the results of laboratory investigations can alter medical practice radically. Unfortunately, it is common experience today that reading contemporary medical and scientific journals is not a routine among physicians. Education for many doctors stopped with commencement.

The Importance of Individuals

One of the purposes of this study is to stress the importance of the individual as the harbinger of change. Many of the doctors I discussed were confident that, in their vision for the future, changes in medical practice, or in the social order or in government were necessary for the health of the people. The entire reform movement of the nineteenth century was based upon the necessity for change so that life would be better for the dispossessed, for the sick, for the ignorant and the abused. From the granting of the degree of doctor of medicine to a woman to the prevention of lead poisoning among factory workers, or from the attempts to clean up tenement living to the introduction of social workers to hospital staffs, we read the story of individuals who responded to what they saw with confidence in their assertion of what was the right course to follow for the health of the people.

These doctors offer us models, not necessarily of persons to be blindly imitated, but as men and women who acted on their experiences after they interpreted the meaning of those experiences for themselves and for others. A pervasive characteristic of these persons is their introspective appraisal of their observations, and their subsequent decision to act upon that appraisal. Some of them ran into significant opposition, but persisted in their conviction of the correctness of their interpretations.

Another aspect of the development of these doctors is their struggle to maintain an open mind to both what they saw and what they learned. It is important for the physician to be awake to the constant flux of apparent facts - some correct and some not so - that fills our sources of information. We must be very careful in our use of the word *know* when we speak about our current beliefs concerning cause and effect and about treatments of diseases. Even a limited study of our history of medicine reveals an astounding number of false assumptions and erroneous conclusions. Medical history is replete with the most absurd and unbelievable narratives of science and of personal behavior. The absolute confidence of the best physicians - Benjamin Rush and his students - in bleeding remains one of the most inconceivable examples. The confidence of so many persons in Thomsonianism, Mesmerism, and the other alternative therapies of the nineteenth century raises questions to this day when the presence of descendents of these practices still speak to some of the failures of orthodox medicine.

Another lesson from our study of history is the need to separate the two mental exercises of *describing* and *explaining.* Perhaps the most important lesson of the past for us is to distinguish between characterizing what we see in our studies and interpreting what we think it means and does. The past history of the sciences is filled with an amazing number of "facts" that bewilder the mind when we consider that they were firmly believed: the earth is flat; the sun revolves around the earth; yellow fever is caused by a miasma in the air; bleeding and purging cure pneumonia; climate is a decisive factor in both the cause and the cure of many diseases. The list is, unfortunately, almost endless.

But we must be very cautious in criticizing the proponents of these theories; they were educated and thoughtful persons carefully examining the evidence they had and then attempting to carry out a very familiar human enterprise: explain what we see. We are rarely satisfied with mere description; we want to explain the whys and the wherefores of experiment. It is not enough to tell what we find in our work. We often feel compelled to explain what it means. The results of this need to explain have had many unfortunate consequences in medicine. A review of the treatments offered for diseases over the many centuries is distressing. All kinds of herbal remedies, electrical stimulations, lotions and potions, and snake oils have been confidently promoted as curative of a wide variety of illnesses. And not only by what we might call 'quacks.' Many of the outstanding physicians of their time were convinced of the rightness of their prescriptions. This is a sober reminder for us of our human propensity to explain the unknowable and therefore to know what to do.

Medical Education

The nineteenth century, as I noted, was a time when medical education was at an all-time low. The proliferation of proprietary schools that offered minimal education and no clinical or laboratory experience provided a phenomenal over-supply of incompetent physicians. The practice of medicine was poorly paid, was held in disrespect as a profession, and was a hazard to the sick. The education of doctors in the colonial period had been by apprenticeship; a young man of promise would, by legal contract, become a clerk-handyman-student of a local physician for a number of years, gradually learning the tools of the trade until he was deemed capable of going into practice. By the 1830s this system was displaced by the proprietary schools and the decline of medical education in America began.

The results of this shift in education were several. Henry S. Pritchett, in his Introduction to the Flexner Report of 1910, described these results.

(1) For twenty-five years past there has been an enormous over-production of uneducated and ill trained medical practitioners. This has been in absolute disregard of the public welfare....Taking the United States as a whole, physicians are four or five times as numerous in proportion to population as in older countries like Germany.

(2) Over-production of ill trained men is due in the main to the existence of a very large number of commercial schools....

(3) ...Many universities desirous of apparent educational completeness have annexed medical schools without making themselves responsible either for the standards of the professional schools or for their support....

(5) A hospital under complete educational control is as necessary to a medical school as is a laboratory of chemistry or pathology....Trustees of hospitals, public and private, should therefore go to the limit of their authority in opening hospital wards to teaching,...[1]

By the time of this report changes were apparent in several medical schools that would alter both the training of doctors and the public image of their skills and importance.

Abraham Flexner, in Chapter I of his 1910 Report to the Carnegie Foundation, described the decline in medical education beginning in the 1820s with the separation of medical schools from university and hospital connections. He documented the astounding proliferation of proprietary schools:

First and last, the United States and Canada have in little more than a century produced four hundred and fifty-seven medical schools, many, of course, short-lived, and perhaps fifty still-born....Illinois, prolific mother of thirty-nine medical colleges, still harbors in the city of Chicago fourteen;...[2]

The wave of commercial expansion that swept through the United States in the second half of the nineteenth century did not exclude even university-related medical schools. Those at Harvard, Yale, and Pennsylvania remained quite detached from the academic structure of the university, hiring and firing, and dispensing of fees in indiscriminate and irresponsible ways. Over the years, various schools had attempted reforms, as did the medical profession itself when it organized into an Association in 1846. But these reforms were slow in being realized. Even the importation of the stethoscope and the microscope from Europe took years to become recognized parts of medical education.

By the 1880s laboratory sciences were becoming recognized as necessary parts of medical education; students began to seek out schools that both required some college education and skills in languages, and also offered clinical and laboratory training in addition to didactic lectures. In 1878 a laboratory was established at the College of Physicians and Surgeons (Columbia University) by Francis Delafield, and a pathology laboratory was opened at Bellevue Hospital by William H. Welch.[3] Twenty years earlier, Northwestern University had initiated a three-year graded course and, as I described earlier,

Harvard achieved control of its medical department in the last quarter of the century under the presidency of Charles W. Eliot. By 1901 Harvard required a college degree for admission. But the major force for reconstruction of medical education in the United States was created in Baltimore in 1893 with the establishment of the Johns Hopkins School of Medicine. In the words of Flexner,

> This was the first medical school in America of genuine university type, with something approaching adequate endowment, well equipped laboratories conducted by modern teachers, devoting themselves unreservedly to medical investigation and instruction, and with its own hospital, in which the training of physicians and the healing of the sick harmoniously combine to the advantage of both....It has finally cleared up the problem of standards and ideals; and its graduates have gone forth in small bands to found new establishments or to reconstruct old ones.[4]

The original clinical faculty of the medical school would become renowned as progenitors of a new American medicine, innovators who brought the renaissance to its realized potential: William Osler physician-in chief, William S. Halsted, surgeon-in-chief, William H. Welch, chief of pathology, and Howard A. Kelly, head of gynecology. Harvey Cushing, resident in surgery under Halsted, would become a leading neurosurgeon and biographer of Osler.

William Osler

As a final example of a person whose influence upon the education and training of physicians was outstanding - perhaps unequaled in our history - I will present a brief note on William Osler (1849-1919). His life and work are the subjects of numerous biographies and papers that eulogize him, often to the point of labeling him as the greatest physician in his century, if not in all of history. Rather than detailing his life and work, I will speak to some characteristics of that life that are important for me and for many other physicians. Osler was a prolific writer on a variety of topics. He wrote the outstanding textbook of medicine for his time; he wrote numerous articles on medical practice, on pathological studies, and on the figures in the past that were models for his own life. He wrote numerous essays on the moral, philosophical and practical aspects of the practice of medicine. It is this latter category that remains a source for introspection and self-evaluation for many physicians to this day. On graduating from the

Johns Hopkins School of Medicine we were presented with a copy of his classic collection of essays, *Aequanimitas With Other Addresses.*

Osler was born in rural Canada, the eighth child of an Anglican minister. He was educated at Trinity College School, briefly attended Toronto School of Medicine - a proprietary school - and went on to get his degree in medicine from McGill University in 1872. At McGill he began his long term interest in the study of pathology, devoting many hours to performing autopsies. He was convinced of the absolute necessity of a first-hand knowledge of pathology if one were to be a competent physician. Osler studied abroad in England, Berlin, and Vienna in the years 1873-74, returning to McGill to teach physiology, pathology, resume his interest in comparative zoology, start a Journal Club, and be appointed a physician to the Montreal General Hospital. In 1884 he accepted the position of chair of clinical medicine at Pennsylvania. Not interested in a general private practice of medicine, Osler devoted much of his time to teaching students and staff. He continued his extensive autopsy studies.

In 1889 Osler left Philadelphia for Baltimore to become physician-in-chief. It was here that his contributions to medicine were fully realized. Osler established the clinical clerkship program for medical students, a system where each student is assigned patients to care for under the supervision of the attending and house staffs. This is the best teaching tool for students, and contributed to the rapid rise of the medical school to its position of eminence. The second innovation of Osler was the creation of the residency program where trained and carefully selected physicians were placed in charge of sections of the medical department and were responsible to Osler for both patient care and teaching. They were called residents because they lived in the hospital. This position drew physicians from across the country to improve their training.

In 1905 Osler, wearied by his duties at Hopkins, accepted the chair of Regius Professor of Medicine at Oxford. This was not a stressful position, and he enjoyed the delights of the University and had ample opportunities for study and writing. Osler died in 1919 of pneumonia. Charles S. Bryan, in his 1997 study, *Osler: Inspirations from a Great Physician,* described Osler as

the most famous and influential physician of the early twentieth century. His life can be seen in brief as the fulfillment of two dreams. As a young man he determined to become a great teacher of clinical medicine. His 1892 textbook, *The Principles and Practice of Medicine,* set a new standard and greatly advanced scientific medicine....[H]e then set out...to reconcile the emerging new medical science with the old humanities. His unique blend of clinical competence, easy familiarity with the liberal arts, energy, charisma, and idealism made him something of a symbol of humanism in medicine for physicians and laypersons alike.[5]

There are several aspects of his life - personal and professional - to be found in his writings that are important to me.

1. While a student at McGill Osler read a sentence by Thomas Carlyle that he quoted (actually misquoted) in a 1913 lecture to Yale students. Osler said, "I picked up a volume of Carlyle, and on the page I opened there was the familiar sentence, *'Our main business is not to see what lies dimly at a distance, but to do what lies clearly at hand.'*"[6] Osler went on in the talk to discuss what he called, *Life in day-tight compartments.* His proposal to his listeners and readers was to focus on the work of this day. The past was the past and the future was yet to make itself known. By concentration on immediate tasks and responsibilities we can accomplish goals not previously thought possible.

2. There is a resource to be had in the writings of authors who can instruct us: poets, playwrights, novelists, essayists and the Bible can add immeasurably to our sense of self and our vision of our world and of our tasks in it. Osler was a renowned bibliophile and collector of books that he not only read, but knew.

3. We would do well to live a simple life with good habits firmly entrenched, habits that set moral standards for our behavior before the time of trial makes itself known. Osler called *work* an essential act for us that determines us. We are to think through who we would become and then work toward that goal.

4. The practice of medicine will require constant study and education in the new scientific determinants of diagnosis and treatment. Collegiality and conversation are crucial to good practice. Osler deplored the "lock and key" type of laboratory, convinced that we are compelled to share what we know and what we have learned.

In the concluding chapter of his 1999 book, *William Osler: A Life in Medicine,* Michael Bliss summed up his appraisal of this memorable doctor.

If there was any undertone of sadness in a happy and wonderfully successful life, it flowed from Osler's understanding that there is no final escape from the oblivion of the grave and the dead house.

He did escape intellectually, moving backwards and forwards through history and communing with the dead through reading and memory and acts of commemoration. In the world of the living, he used time to the fullest....Osler did not fear death, but he understood the shortness and precariousness of life....His special satisfaction and enduring example came in the quest and camaraderie of healing, struggling to realize the gospel of helping to make it possible for men and women and children to have more time and less pain. This was and is a life well lived.[7]

It has been a long century from Jacob Bigelow to William Osler. But it was a time when certain physicians saw what was present to them, attempted to understand what they saw, and worked to effect some change in their environs. These doctors offer us models for studying our world, both personally and professionally, so that we might be able to contribute to the goal of increasing lifetimes and reducing the pains we suffer in them.

---

[1]Pritchett, Henry S., "Introduction," *Medical Education in the United States and Canada,* by Abraham Flexner, Boston, The Merrymount Press, 1910, x-xi.
[2]Flexner, Abraham, Ibid., 6.
[3]Ibid., 11.
[4]Ibid., 12.
[5]Bryan, Charles S., *Osler: Inspirations from a Great Physician,* New York, Oxford University Press, 1997, vii.
[6]Osler, William, *A Way of Life,* Baltimore, Remington-Putnam Book Company, 1932, 19.
[7]Bliss, Michael, *William Osler: A Life in Medicine,* New York, Oxford University Press, 1999, 502.

Index